ALL I NEED IS HERE

Surviving Anxiety and Depression

Nicola Espeut

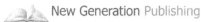

DEDICATION

I would like to dedicate this book to Paul McEvoy, a gentle giant and close friend who took his life in the early part of 2020. I wish I could have let him read it before he died. It might have made a difference.

Table of Contents

ACKNOWLEDGMENTS

I would like to thank my mother for inspiring me to write this book and for always supporting me, and my two brothers Andre and Howard, for their advice and encouragement over the years. Also, to the Julian Campbell Foundation, who persuaded me to start this book sooner than I had planned.

I would also like to thank the Viktor Frankl Institute especially for their work on finding a purpose in life, and getselfhelp.co.uk for their resources.

CHAPTER 1 — COPING WITH ANXIETY

Do not find fault. Find a remedy.
– Henry Ford

I had never imagined that I would be the one to suffer from anxiety. I had always been a happy-go-lucky person, without a worry in the world.

It happened about six months ago when I'd just come out of hospital, and I didn't know for the first time in my life what to do with myself or how to use my time. Previously, I had been peacefully drifting, spending much of my time in libraries or on courses — that seemed to satisfy my needs. I had a decent group of friends, and was social enough not to feel isolated, and still be mentally stimulated. The libraries were local, and the educational pursuits were just how I wanted them to be. I explored and brought back souvenirs, memories, and experiences from outer boroughs, but stayed grounded in North London nevertheless. So yes, when I developed anxiety, I had no idea what to do with myself. I had exhausted several avenues. There were always suggestions about why I didn't try to do this or that. But everything seems impossible when you have acute anxiety, bordering on panic attacks. Even getting to the stage where trying to heal becomes practically impossible.

The best help I received was from a Hypnotherapist. He spurred me on to heal myself and suggested journaling. He also suggested that I should write a book, something I've always wanted to do, but more notably, he reminded me of the importance of managing my time and my emotions. Time management is a way of showing accountability — a method of pictorial justifications of your time and how it's spent. The thing was, going to the library, although a grounding activity for me, offered no quantification of time spent. This is what I felt was lacking in my life — a way to show myself how to live life to the fullest! The pain I felt was excruciating. There were days where I would do nothing but lay on my bed, looking at what needed to be done and not having the energy or courage to do anything about it. When I needed support, the first thing I would do was pray and have a talk with God. And God didn't want us to have a spirit of fear. In fact, this poem says it better than I could have penned myself:

<u>Our deepest fear</u>
By Marianne Williamson

Our deepest fear is not that we are inadequate

Our deepest fear is that we are powerful beyond measure

It is our light, not our darkness that most frightens us

We ask ourselves

"Who am I to be brilliant, gorgeous, talented fabulous?"

Actually, who are you not to be? You are a child of God

Your playing small does not serve the world

There's nothing enlightened about shrinking

So that other people won't feel insecure around you.

We are all meant to shine, as children do

We are born to manifest the glory of God

That is within us.

It's not just in some of us; it's in everyone

And as we let our light shine, we unconsciously

Give other people permission to do the same.

As we're liberated from our own fear,

Our presence automatically liberates others.

Thus, I began to appreciate that it is our light, not our darkness, that we are stifling. Our darkness is a side of us that needs to be tamed and chained down with a ball. It does not serve us, nor does it relent if you dwell on it.

Courage to go through the darkness — the quagmire, as I call it — is not you but is part of you for now, as you have not confronted or challenged it. It takes the courage of a roaring lion to ask for help in these situations. Often, we feel that we'd be bringing the other person down with us. Although it is possible, I go by this advice and say that you are responsible for your own happiness. No one can make you feel unhappy if you do not give them that power or permission.

During this journey, I have had many conversations

with God. I was wishfully trying to calm the gastric chemicals, the heart-burn, the tension, and the headaches. One thing that I constantly repeated was, Jesus, have mercy on me. I said this repetitively about ten times in a trying-to-calm-myself-down kind of manner. When the pain was so apparent, and the cause was just the inability to do anything, it felt like I needed a thunderbolt to propel me towards taking action.

It's relatively easy to lose yourself and slump into inactivity, and it starts with an untidy home. Sooner or later, you stop caring about your meals, and then before you know it, you do not want to go out. There are too many chores to do. You do not want to stay in to do them or come back to find them. That is when I repeated another prayer – "God, give me the courage to do what I find difficult. God, render all obstacles obsolete from before me now. I cannot live without you in my life. So that I'm immersed in you, please be the light that guides my path."

It's astonishing how simple tasks during the day become the most significant achievements of the day — making your bed, putting away the laundry — is considered a big accomplishment. Organizing a healthy lunch or dinner makes you feel better instantly. I believe anxiety comes from the lack of fuel to the brain. Your brain just simply fails to cope with minimal life stressors, and a small thing like breaking a plate becomes a huge deal.

Some people suggest distracting yourself. What better way to do that than making yourself something nutritional to eat or organizing your wardrobe, so you do not have to worry about what to wear daily?

Now, what do you do when an anxiety attack is coming at you full throttle?

The symptoms:
- Sweaty hands
- Shortness of breath
- Heartburn
- Shaking
- Sweating
- Nervousness
- Tension
- Worry
- Laziness
- Lack of motivation
- Irritability
- Rapid heart rate
- Twitching tremors
- Daytime fatigue
- Pessimism
- Disorientation and dizziness

The triggers:
- Getting out of bed
- Going to work
- Going to social occasions
- Finding a new address
- Going on a journey
- Meeting new people
- Going on a holiday
- Talking to people on the phone

- Talking in groups
- Starting a new course
- Starting a new job
- Leaving the house
- Cooking the dinner
- Getting shopping in

Whatever the symptoms or whatever the triggers, over time I have found a few things that help me cope in these situations. Start by doing some breathwork, just take a few deep breaths — the deeper, the better. If you have not already planned to start your day with some sort of physical activity such as push-ups, Yoga, Tai chi, Pilates, running, walking, or cycling, you should plan one now. A combination of these activities and incorporation of them into your day would work wonders for you.

Next, keep a diary for yourself. In it, write not only what you have done but what you want to do, and plan it so that your weeks are not always empty.

It's better to have activities lined-up beforehand so that you do not have lots of free time to worry and get anxious about being idle.

Plan a healthy time or a fun time to do the things that you enjoy at least once every two weeks, if you cannot do it every week. Also, put goals into your diary. Finish a course, a piece of art, some knitting or sewing project, write the first 1,000 words of a book. These are all tangible goals you can hold onto so that when you are fretting later on in life about not doing anything, these could serve as concrete evidence that you have been doing something. Also, engaging in such activities keep you active, that's why planning beforehand is so vital. It will give you a chance to discover new things and will help you stay fit. It enables the mind to wander off to more pleasant destinations, instead of ruminating.

As soon as anxiety takes over, you cannot help but think about how you have not achieved a certain goal in life and how it has become increasingly difficult to do so. You will keep thinking about everything that has put you down and held you back from achieving your goals. This kind of thought process is immobilizing — though it does not mean it cannot be stopped. It all starts with the first word being written, and the first step you take before you start running again. So, at this point, it's time for another chat, and what better than the title of this book.

All I need is here.

I discovered this beautiful phrase whilst on a camping holiday in England. At one of camp's workshops, we were encouraged to sing this song — all I need is here, all I need is here, all I need is here — such a comforting thought.

We have the innate ability to be self-sufficient. It reminds us that whatever it is that we need, we can find it here within ourselves or close by. What I found helpful was speaking to someone about my problems. If you want to call a helpline to talk your heart out, you need to make that call with the belief that someone is always there for you 24 hours a day, 365 days a year, at the other end of the line, ready to help you. You just need to believe in that tiny amount of goodness — believe that it exists in the world — and make that call.

Before you second guess yourself and make a rash decision, you need to talk to someone —to discuss whatever issue — just make that call.

There is no point in wallowing and drowning in a pool of worries. It is so easy to slip but it's just a small setback. When there is even a little doubt, we second guess ourselves and question ourselves and then we start spiralling into fear and anxiety, which leads to depression and disease. The trick is to remember a verse just as worry and doubt start to enter the mind.

Do not be anxious about anything, but in everything, by prayer and petition with thanksgiving, present your requests to God and the peace of God — it surpasses all understanding and will quieten your heart and your mind in Christ Jesus (Philippians 4:6, 7)

By petition and prayer, present your requests in front of your Lord. It's nice to think that there is something that you can petition. At times, it's good to add the thanksgiving first — we should thank God for the times that we might not remember because that schedule would have changed magnanimously. Once I began my days differently, I needed to learn to have faith; faith is something that I wanted to quantify before showing examples of what I have achieved through faith, but it is possible to measure it especially on the days where you think you have no one with you. Prayers keep you alive, but that's why it's good to have a diary to remember what it is you have asked for.

Now, let's get back to tackling anxiety head-on. When do the doubts and fears set in? And what can be done about it? I found that doubts and fears come into my mind as soon as I get home or at times when I feel I am going to be on my own again. Doubts start in the form of a question — they commonly start like this; what are you going to do with your life? Followed swiftly by, where are you going? Then, how will you find the means? Normal questions for most people but relentless for me, to the point that I have questioned my own sanity several times.

It's amazing how the question 'what are you going to do with your life?' Stirs such fear and anxiety. I consider myself lucky that there are some options at my disposal. I guess I have another 25 years if I am fortunate. So, surely I should be planning what I want to do with my life, instead of worrying about it. Try rephrasing the question like this   what would you like to do with your life if you had the option of doing anything you wanted to do? Where have you not visited yet, but would like to visit? Think of a place, maybe somewhere of historical interest, why do you want to go there? What do you want to see?

It's really important how you phrase the question and what your answers are. For ages, my response used to be — I do not know what to do with my life. I did want to do something though, I just didn't know what! One day, I got what I call a 'lightning seed moment', when it finally occurred to me that I wasn't all that hopeless and acknowledged that I was good at what I do. Either that or things that I did in my past made me proud today. It might take others to show you this, but by listening to this input, sometimes you can acknowledge your brilliance without letting your ego run amok.

Recovery is like being in a tunnel for four months. This

is essentially a time where you need the lightning seeds to light up the walls around you. As this place is pitch black, you may not want to go out at all. You are despondent — you have too much time on your hands and you are not coping with the basics of healthy food, good sleep, and exercise — you find it hard to concentrate. There are days when you want to call out to friends, but they have moved on with their lives and cannot be there for you when you need them the most.

So, you need to develop a coping mechanism and not present yourself as overly needy. It's nice to have an empathetic friend who is there to support you during your difficult times. Sometimes, you need those cuddles or someone who can wipe your tears away. I was exactly this person for many people. For many years I was the strong one and people would often share their woes with me. But, I guess that along the way, their worries became a burden on me, and I let them affect me too much. In the end, I think the weight of everything caused my mind to implode. There is only so much one person can take. I felt like I was stuck in a rut, but what's worse is this feeling was compacted because I was in the tunnel — it is in these moments that you must remember the lightning seeds that you cannot live without. The darkness is like a quagmire, where the demons tell you that you are not worth anything, and freely reside with all the insecurities and doubts you harbour. This is where loneliness takes its roots and engulfs you in its darkness. It makes you worry and so self-doubt creeps in, feeding on your diminished self-esteem and low confidence. All together, as fiendish friends, these add to the darkness in that quagmire. No wonder you seem outnumbered. These are the demons that engulf you, surround you, and eventually consume you, so that there is nothing left of you.

Where there is a worry, there is fear — where there is fear, there is sadness, loneliness, doubt(s), and insecurities. This is not a good building block for an individual. Imagine that this is all the personality that you have — it consists of mud, the tunnel, and the quagmire. As a result, it starves you of inspiration, creative genius, motivation, life juice, connectivity, and hope, leaving you empty and numb. But, if you remember your lightning seeds, they lead you to think of a hobby, something you like doing.

In hard times, try to think of them quickly!

It can be that or something you were good at. It can be of a place you liked visiting; think of going there again when you feel better. But it's better to think of a craft or something that you can do immediately or by yourself. It will work, even if it is simply playing an instrument. Anything that takes you away from what it is that you are feeling. This way, you can feel that you have accomplished something.

Repeat things you enjoy doing when you are in the tunnel, as this is the place where you are most vulnerable and the likelihood of self-torment is greater.

I had a Medusa-like image that constantly berated me, telling me that I was good for nothing. It sabotaged any progress I made. It continuously talked me down, eroded my confidence, and made me feel repressed, degenerated, unable to accomplish anything, stagnated, fearful and obsolete, with no future.

Tackling Medusa was difficult as she was always present, willing to spill the beans of my life. It is disheartening not to be courageous and not to have the momentum to move forward — she was always there in front of me and stopped any progression, even any positive actions or thoughts. She was pushing me into the depths of the tunnel, the quagmire, the place from where there was no return. She would show her ugly head frequently as if to repeat the same woeful messages continuously, enforcing the same doom and gloom that makes one too paralyzed to do anything. Again, this is where you need to be nurtured and encouraged: the lightning seeds. All I need is here!

How they manifest in these times is a glimmer of hope. When you feel paralyzed and have nowhere to turn to, you need something to get you through the day and a glimmer of hope can be the best reassurance at this time. With good news and reviewed thoughts, you may relieve the tension in your body by taking a few deep breaths.

All I need is here — now imagine a white light over your head, and close your eyes. Imagine this light heals, and that it can enter your body. It starts in your head and travels through the rest of your body slowly, releasing all trauma and fear, healing you gently. Imagine this light reaching your feet, going to the tips of your hands, immersing you in the comfort and knowledge that you are on the route to being healed completely.

All I need is here — now heal the tension related to anxiety. It can heal you from the shadows of the negative outer voices — all I need is *here*. Make this your mantra and keep chanting it. All I need is here, all I need is here. Go back to the light. Let it finish its work. Working from the top of the body, right down to the toes, everything that is touched by the light will be healed. This is the same method for other minor ailments. Imagine that you are in a room full of people, and they are listening attentively to your every word, imagine that you have the confidence to speak effortlessly, and your audience receives you wholeheartedly. Imagine not questioning or wondering what you are going to say next, just enjoy the stimulating conversation when you are being listened to and heard.

It all goes back to — all I need is here.

Feel the tension leave your body as you look towards the healing light. Let it immerse you and heal your body of all tension and all anxiety. Ask for the soothing light to enter all parts of the body that require healing.

Let all your fears subside; fear about what you are going to do next, fear about future goals and ambitions, fears about your present situation. Let them all subside and return to the healing light that erases all those fearful shadows from your mind. All I need is here, to remain calm and believe in a fearless existence — one where all your needs are met, one where fear does not take a hold of your life.

CHAPTER 2 — LEARNING CONFIDENCE

The only thing we have to fear is fear itself.
— *Oscar Wilde*

Have confidence in yourself, build this resource like a muscle, practice — be more confident every day. Do things to show confidence. A head full of fears leaves no space for dreams. Worry does nothing but steal your joy and keep you busy doing nothing. Stop all the negative thoughts you have about yourself, such as believing you will never be able to write a book or that you will never be good enough to change careers.

With all the 'you will never' thoughts, followed by the 'never can dos', it's important to shed some light on them because they often belong to the same list.

Here are some of my popular ones:

- You will never own a house
- You will never find a partner
- You will never get a job
- You will never find new friends
- You will never enjoy your life
- You will never amount to anything
- You will never find your passion
- You will never lose weight
- You will never go on holiday

These are some of the self-limiting thoughts that I had daily. This is what I had to deal with every passing day, sometimes even before I got up in the morning. In some cases, as soon as I was up and running, a stream of negative self-talk would take over my brain, which does not, of course, serve me or anyone else.

The key to success is to do more of the things that work and less of the things that do not work. Part of the not-working-scenario is the negative self-talk that just leads to a sort of mental paralysis, and you have to find a way to circumvent it. For every negative question, there has to be a positive alternative. To this end, you need to determine your 'brand' of negative self-talk. I have listed mine to help you write your own. As soon as this is established, you need to de-establish it. You are your worst enemy. Every time you think of something negative, which might be often, you have to replace it with a positive phrase, and if anyone you know adds to your feeling of worthlessness, it's better not to be around them. This is why you need to surround yourself with positive people and experiences. Anytime you feel yourself slipping into feelings of insignificance, be prepared to have a new strategy.

So, for example, I do not think I am good enough to find a new partner. Firstly, be the best partner for yourself so you can stand alone. Be resourceful and self-contained, then go and attract a new partner. Never say you are not good enough for someone else. Be good enough for yourself and let that standard be sufficient. Then you are ready to go into the dating arenas brimming with self-confidence.

Also, remember to continue to take care of yourself; as in your appearance, your clothes, they should be clean and tidy, and you should be clean. Make an effort with your hair and outward appearance. Never let this slip. You could be anywhere and run into anyone. It's best not to look like a knackered heap. Take pride in your appearance and make an effort.

How you present yourself says a lot about you and your self-worth. Go for regular hairdresser appointments, wear clothes that suit you and your personality. Try a new look, but make sure you are comfortable. Get help from friends and family. Say you are trying something different — you want to get a new hairstyle that says success, that says achievements, that says you want to attract a partner in your life. Also ask for tips, things that might help you succeed in your aims.

Consider it a job interview, but do not slip back into a negative mindset that you will never get a job. Is it important to know why you want a job? Is it going to take over your life? Are you a workaholic? Do you want it just for social interaction, or do you want it just to pay the bills? Be aware of what you want the job for and try to meet your needs in other ways. If it's just social interaction you want, you may be able to achieve this by joining a group doing exercises, or a hobby like joining an art class.

A job is not the be-all and end-all of life. You must learn not to think in absolutes. All-or-nothing thinking is not helpful. Being a workaholic, I understand the importance of being distinctive about your work-life balance. Work is sometimes just a means to an end; it's not everything, and it shouldn't be the most important part of your life. You need balance in everything.

Besides, it helps to be a more rounded individual, having interests outside of work helps to combat stress and stops you from overthinking. You can easily fall into the all or nothing mindset at work, so you need to do everything you can to have a better work-life balance.

One huge problem with anxiety is stress, which can be a result of the scales tipping more one way than the other when it comes to the work-life balance, but stressing out about these things is futile. To level out the work-life balance, it's important to consider what stressors you have related to work. The aim is to take on a work position with the least amount of stress on you, while remembering that this could be a different position for someone else. What *your* stressors are, are not the same for other people — stress triggers are very personal.

So, identify your stressors and carefully assign numbers to them, or asterisks for that matter. Then, identify where and when you are feeling them, let's say its meeting new people in a job. A scale of 1-10 should help you determine how it makes you feel, one being awful, ten being excellent, and rate your performance in every part of your job. State what you like best and rate these too — and to add some positivity, asterisk your favourite parts of the job. Lastly, look for finding the equivalent of this outside a job.

Now get back to daily living. What if when you wake up, the first thought you have is, 'I feel so lonely.' How does that affect your day and your level of anxiety? What if you have nothing planned for the day; no job and no interactions. This could be pretty damaging for you since your self-esteem will be at an all-time low, and your level of anxiety will be high. The best course of action — instead of staying indoors — is to go out somewhere where you can meet people or at least have the opportunity to meet and greet people. I say — take a bus, go into town, and go to a coffee shop or the library. It could be anywhere. Wherever a group of people gather, join them! That's where you need to start. That's how you tackle anxiety. The feeling of loneliness is surprisingly heavy when coupled with anxiety.

Feelings of loneliness tied up with feelings of abandonment, losing connections with your surroundings, and your community — all of these, when combined, make a recipe for disaster.

Losing touch, or even being out of reality, sometimes is also a common sign. All of these symptoms should be dealt with as soon as possible before they worsen. Drawing into your reserves to make yourself happy is good enough, and a lot of things can be done privately, of course. However, having a regular rapport with people, especially at set times, helps to build a routine and reduce anxiety. Loneliness is one of the biggest triggers for anxiety. The feeling of being alone with your sulky self, combined with the feelings that 'you cannot get any help,' 'you have no support', and 'you are trapped', all stem from this loneliness cloud. This crippling loneliness cloud can surround you, engulf you, and numb you into an anxious state.

What do you do about these feelings? Are they contagious? Does someone warn you about them?
The feeling of anxiety is heightened when this cloud of loneliness surrounds you, almost suffocating you. So, as always, it is important to breathe; breathe deep, and let your breath out. Repeat this so that you can ward off the cloud of loneliness — breathe out, take in a

huge breath, and breathe out again. By doing this, you have altered your heartbeat and stopped sinking into that gloomy, shallow thought.

If you learn to breathe correctly, this will calm you down when you start feeling anxious. It will help with the supply of oxygenated blood to the brain and will allow you to think more rationally.

Another tip is to set up an exercise routine. Anxiety feeds on free time, so the more you can plan things for your day, the better. And remember, we only need 7 hours of sleep a day.

The first thought when you wake up is crucial as it sets the tone for the day. For example, what am I going to do today? Is better than, what am I going to do with my entire life? It's good to get yourself a diary and write down things that you are doing every day. This alleviates stress and anxiety, and enables you to plan more things in to your schedule.

While it is good to relax, spare time can cause problems, so try to think of activities that you normally like to do, for instance; swimming, visiting a museum, going for a walk, skating, horse-riding or playing tennis. List them in your diary so that even if you do not do any of these, at least the options are there for another time. It is important to make the best of your time. Whether it is filling in a personal blog or playing an instrument, if you document it, at least you know how your time is going to be spent.

The only thing that remains is to find an activity that you enjoy — and do more of that. If it's a physical activity and gets you out of the house into the countryside, that is even better. Take in the fresh air to heighten the senses.

The more you are out doing things, the better it is for you, as it counters anxiety head-on.

What I also find useful is setting alarms on your phone as reminders — for example, in the form of a living diary to plug you into the day. If you are like me, the first thought in the morning is aimed towards discouraging you, so set the alarm for something fun. For instance, when you wake up, let it be your favourite music that rings in your ears, or why not select a joke to break the mood when things are too dark and dismal? There is always an answer and everyone has a different one.

I also frequently turned to the Bible in my hours of despair, and the words inspired me greatly. I thought I should put Psalm 23 in here.

The Lord is my shepherd; I lack nothing.
He makes me lie down in green pastures,
He leads me beside quiet waters
He refreshes my soul.
He guides me along the right paths for his name's sake.
Even though I walk through the darkest valley,
I will fear no evil,
For you are with me;
Your rod and your staff
They comfort me.
You prepare a table before me
In the presence of my enemies.
You anoint my head with oil
My cup overflows.
Surely your goodness and love will follow me
All the days of my life,
And I will dwell in the house of the Lord forever.

Though it might feel like you have to walk through the valley of death, a place of extreme despair and anguish, that it is the worst scenario of your life, so never forget that there is always light at the end of the tunnel.

Without fear, what could you accomplish?

I have had some sort of anxiety my whole life. Whether it is a fear of going out or fear of staying in, you name it. Yet, I achieved many milestones in my youth. It's just that now that I am older, I feel as if those milestones need to be more frequent as I try to quantify and justify what I am doing with my life now.

Usually, in the mornings, my biggest fear is what I am going to do today and I do not start to feel better until mid-afternoon. Then it gets worse again as the evening draws closer, and I just keep thinking what I am going to do next. This constant questioning makes me feel uneasy for the most part. Interestingly, it is quite a useful thing to know what you are doing for the day. It is a good thing — it's kind of training you to get a job with a schedule. What's better is that you adapt to your new lifestyle, if you are without a job, so that your days can be filled and be more fulfilling.

You do not need a job to make your life feel fulfilled — but it helps — when you follow the simple rules of having a job and function. If you do have a job, it will help you immensely with your wellbeing.

We have already suggested some things you can do first thing in the morning if your anxiety hits you then, but let's look at some other things we can do, too. I try to start the day with at least 20 press-ups. I do not always do them, but to start the day with press-ups gets the blood pumping through the body, and it's a great way to start the day. The next idea is to have a good breakfast and spend time making something wholesome and nutritious. Always have a large drink with it. This can include water, fruit juices, smoothies and cups of tea. It all helps us to hydrate. Have a good, long shower to clean your body. Give it a hard scrub in the mornings, and wash your hair if you have time. Put on some fresh, clean clothes and add a scent; it always makes you feel better.

Get into a routine with your clothes so that you rotate them and always have clean clothes to put on. Coordinate your clothes — know what you are going to be wearing for the day and then lay them out in advance so that you are not running around in the morning, not knowing what to wear. It's also a good idea to plan outfits for a week, since it keeps you stress-free later on. It will curb your anxiety immensely and enable you to get out of that door a little bit quicker than usual.

And that is the object of the game, to be honest — anything that helps you get out of the house and into the fresh air works. Anything that helps stop the pangs of anxiety from consuming you at home, works. It allows you to make a movement or shift your thinking patterns and helps you start the day with a purpose. It's an effort that puts anxiety at bay.

It's also a good idea to write your to-do list for the next day the night before. Keep your diary by your side, and write notes constantly. It does not matter if they are copious. The more you write, the more grounded you are day-to-day. You can break the day into segments and write something for each segment of the day. Say, 7-11a.m., 11a.m.-3p.m., 3-7p.m., or 7-10 p.m. — anything that works. Whether you are planning a meal or making a phone call, make sure you are occupied at these times of the day, and if you are not, write that down as well, there is no reason why you should not relax at any time in a whole day. There is no reason why you shouldn't start making use of these hours in the day. It is also great to write. I always resort to writing when I feel like I am going to be free for the next few hours.

As I mentioned before, plan your days like workdays. Decide what times you like to undertake the core activities. Work out for yourself whether you are an early bird or a night owl. If you find it easier getting down to work in the morning, organize your days so that you have most of it done in the morning — plan to unwind in the evening or add in a social event to attend.

Whatever you do, try to strike a healthy balance between work and play, one that works for you. You must have designated playtime. Without it, there is an imbalance. Playtime helps with your anxiety. Having a conversation helps ease any stress that has been building up and allows you to unwind; some even say it's better than therapy. Just make sure that you add this important time to your diary, and besides, all work and no play makes for a very unhappy individual.

So, what happens when you wake up? You have no routine, your anxiety levels are at an all-time high, you do not know whether to stay in or go out, you feel awful, and you do not know what issue to tackle first. Well, the first thing to do as a matter of routine is to make sure that you have breakfast. This will start getting the cerebral juices flowing. After that, do your morning exercise. Actually, it's better to do your exercise before and then go for breakfast. Interestingly, exercising immediately after getting out of bed reduces your anxiety levels.

After breakfast, take the time to start writing in your diary. There is always something that you need to do — whether it's just getting the food from the supermarket or routine stuff — there is always something. Remember that routine is essential, especially with exercise. If you really cannot think of anything to do in the day, take yourself to a coffee shop with a note pad and a pen, and let the outdoors inspire you. Let the collection of people that surround you inspire you to plan something further on in the day for yourself.

Remember that many people around you are doing precisely the same. You are coming out from the indoors and working on something or another, but just doing it in a company of others this time. Now, take some time to visualize what it is that you want from the day. How prepared are you for it? Can you stay out all day, or do you have to be back at a given time? If it is your spare time, what do you like best about being outside? What and where would you go if money and time wasn't an issue? Would you venture, for instance, to another coffee shop further away from the one you usually visit? Or maybe venture somewhere to eat in the daytime? This could be a regular thing so that you are out of your house. Stop by certain shops, and make yourself known to certain places as a regular. Greet people, interact, and be part of life as much as you can. People will begin to notice you once you get out there. Staying indoors throughout the day is not good for anyone. No one gets to see you or know you for the beautiful, loveable, and intelligent person that you are!

So, make it your routine. If you can do things on-the-go, it's all for the better. That means you can be anywhere and get things done. You do not have to be under house arrest. For every symptom, there is an antidote. It's similar to having a buzzing headache, you may try an aspirin or something a little stronger.

If you have anxiety, you have to defeat the inner voices — the negative voices — that always put you down. It's time to put an end to the negative chatter. This endless chatter is defeatist. Its only ambition is to destroy and deflate you in every way possible. Sometimes, it stems straight from fear and this can be spiritual, too. It could mean that you are under a spiritual attack.

So, I suggest that you read Psalm 91 and meditate on its words. And not only that, but Psalm 3 in the morning and Psalm 4 at night. In Psalm 91, it talks about not being afraid and successfully eliminating all fears, that is why it's good to meditate on it. You could try it every half an hour, and it works like aspirin for a headache — it can reprogram your mindset. Whenever you are fearful, you can turn to it, you can carry it on your phone or write it down and carry it in your handbag. This way, you always have it with you. If you read it enough, you will surely be able to memorize it.

The trouble with anxiety is that it masks the true

person inside you. It's almost like you have to step out into the light and reclaim your personality. So, taking off the outer layer of anxiety opens you up to a new way of communicating and that's what you want to achieve by removing the layers. You can find the 'true' you which has been hiding, or been on standby, making your life incomplete. It's like you're waiting in the flanks while the substitute is being called up.

It's so important that, despite how hard it seems, you must try to discover the true you and reveal this to other people; there is nothing laudable about being shy. It does not show your true self or your capabilities, which means you are running at 20% — that's 20% of your personality and your capacity. You are not getting the most from your interactions, and it is obvious.

Sometimes, you may feel anxious from the start of the day. For example, when you are meeting people that you do not know, it can always be a difficult assignment to deal with people head-on. To be free of anxiety, the goal is to make the most of your interactions so you can have a fuller, more wholesome, and authentic life.

CHAPTER 3 — BELIEVE IN YOURSELF

Do not dwell in the past; do not dream of the future;
concentrate the mind on the present moment.
— *Mother Teresa*

There are special techniques that can help you with the start of the day, especially when fear takes hold of you. First, work out how it manifests. If, like me, you are used to getting up and feeling fear straight away — and this has nothing to do with your interactions with people — then this is a serious mindset that you have to conquer in the morning. Anxiety leaves you with a queasy feeling and can make you feel sickly, as well as cause shortness of breath and panic attacks. Feelings of low self-worth soon follow after this.

So yes, it's about turning off the inner voice that tells you that you are not good enough, you won't amount to anything, you are not worthy of attention, and that you shouldn't even exist. This is the self-chatter that you have to learn to re-transpose. Change the inner dialogue so that it is positive. Replace this self-deprecating chatter. Replace it, and those negative thoughts, with positive affirmations. I have included some examples of how you can face the morning's anxieties.

Tell yourself — I am a child gifted into this universe. I have every right to be here. I am loved and am loveable. I choose to focus on things that make me feel good. I am a welcomed child of this universe and I deserve a good life just like everyone else. My thoughts are just a temporary condition. My thoughts are not a reality. The reality is that I am a living, breathing, gorgeous individual who is capable of doing a lot of things. I *can* do this. I *can* do that. I have all the skills inside to enable me to do what I so desire to do. I can remove the shyness that has inhabited me. I can feel better in myself. I can learn to love all parts of myself, equally. I am capable of this type of love. I am a worthy human being; worthy of respect and love. I am assertive and can bring the things I need in life, to me. I know how to attract good things into my life. I can attract like-minded people towards me. I can speak and people are interested in me when I speak, I need not be nervous. I will not let my circumstances define me.

We are all in the gutter, but some of us are looking at the stars.
– Oscar Wilde

Back to positive affirmations. It's important to realize where you are and the things that you have already, rather than the things you have not got. Only, try to be grateful by remembering the things you have. You can keep it simple; it might just be being able to walk, having good eyesight, having good health — these are all things one should be grateful for.

Keep it simple.

While creating an appreciation list, include things like these — having good friends, having a roof over your head, having a meal, trips to the beach or forest, spontaneous picnics. Write them down and learn to memorize them. So that when you are having an off day, apart from your affirmations, you have a reason to be grateful for something. This will greatly reduce anxiety levels.

Another thing that you can do is purchase a pet. It is a known fact that caring for an animal helps reduce tension and stress. Stroking a cat or dog can release tension and has proven to be beneficial for your stress-relieving habits. You can do such things as go for a walk with your dog. It not only takes you out, but it also puts you in the company of animals, who are a great source of stress-relief — worrying about things that might not even happen builds up anxiety and stress. Thinking too far into the future when it isn't necessary also does this.

Your brain presumes things to be worse than they are — often through fear and catastrophizing things. The worst-case scenario might never happen. But the mind-set of negatively thinking all of the time is self-defeating. In the end, there is little movement between point A and point B. Fear immobilizes you, and then the negative feelings catch on, and before than you know it, you wish your life away.

This fear cycle is not sustainable. Sooner or later, you will go into a deep, depressive state because you are stuck in this cycle. Somehow you have to switch off the negative self-talk and the catastrophizing element, which some people take comfort in.

Getting to the stage where you can break the fear cycle is one thing, but the only way you can challenge this is to inject some hope into the future. So whenever you are hell-bent on thinking about something negative, try to introduce something positive in its place — this could be something like your affirmations.

Tell yourself every day that you can do things in your life and make choices for the better — choices that are fulfilling and right for you. You need to tell yourself that you are worthy and deserving of having good things happen to you, and you will make a constant effort to attract these new positive experiences in your life. By letting your mantra be "All I need is here," you're breaking the negative spiral of "I am not enough". Say it when you are making your breakfast in the mornings — I am worthy of this nutrition, it is going to benefit me, it will make me stronger and happier, it is going to fulfil my needs.

Let your mantra of "I am capable of negotiating every aspect of my daily life" affect your very being. Repeat this as internal dialogue — I am worthy of it. I deserve better. I have the right to be happy in all situations. I am courageous. I am honourable. I deserve good things in life. I can make my future into what I dream it to be, I just have to put in the effort. I can rid myself of anxiety and fear by not focusing on the negative aspects of my life. I can always think of positive outcomes from now on, and get rid of the cycle of fear in my life.

The first thing to do is to follow the positive steps in your life.

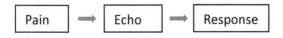

(Copyright Espeut 2021)

Pain = trauma/shock/emotional/ physical pain

Echo = vibrational impact on the body/brain

Response = fight or flight response

One way of looking at depression and anxiety is using the Espeut model. Find out where the pain is entering the body, especially the trigger for it. For example you may develop headaches (pain) as a result of the stress at work *the trigger*. Then establish where in the body you find it (the echo); where is the vibrational impact and how does it manifest? As a headache, stomach ache, muscle tension, etc. Then work out how the body responds (the response).

Does the body or brain try to resist these feelings? Does it make you lethargic? Or does it send alarm signals throughout the body? Such as hypervigilance, trouble focusing or recalling things, and being more emotional than usual. And does this lead to substance abuse or alcohol misuse, as a way of relieving some of these symptoms? Or would you take to relaxation, breathing techniques, meditation or soaking in a bath? (Source unknown internet)

When you come across negative feelings on your path, listen to them, acknowledge that they are harmful, and then dismiss them as unhelpful feelings. Learn to fixate on the positives whenever you experience negative ones. This internal dialogue can help — I am worthy of feeling good, and having nice and pleasant things happen to me in my life. I am worthy of feeling good and healthy with a lovely future to look forward to, and there is a series of good things planned for and established to happen in my life.

There is also a mantra for when you are feeling despondent, low in confidence, or during a panic attack in the street — I can take in breath efficiently and slowly. I am aware of my senses. I connect and am connected to everything in the universe, I am safe, I am loved, and I am enough.

More often than not, it is just fear getting in the way of things. For example, that new job that you do not try for because you think you are not good enough. If you leave your skills dormant enough, they will eventually fail you.

Always keep your skills and approach up to date, instead of thinking about the worst thing that could happen. Always look for the silver lining.

So, when thinking of anything, keep the best outcome in mind. When you wake up in the morning, try visualization. Get yourself a working and unused pen, and plan what it is you want to achieve. Use pictures, words, and phrases, and spend some time on it.

Visualize how you want to see yourself first. Practise being this new person and soon enough, you will start to *be* this new person. Appreciate the new you! Then take the steps you have drawn out for yourself to become the new you.

Change your hair and your clothing style until you feel it suits you. Drop down two sizes to fit into your new clothes. Have a can-do attitude, and volunteer to change things for yourself and your life. There is no better time to start the new you than today! Make positive changes in your lifestyle, changes of habit that will bolster you. Get up earlier in the morning than you have before, and start a cleaning regime. Clean yourself and your environment. Clear your brain of clutter from all your self-limiting beliefs. Take a long, deep breath.

Make it a first to believe in yourself. The thing is that it's only up to you to convince yourself that you are worthy, which is the hardest part. If you do not think that you are worthy, neither will others. So, build up your self-esteem by establishing your worth, and be thankful that every day you get up is a new opportunity to start again.

There are, of course, many things you can do to relieve anxiety. One of them is counting; counting very slowly can relax the mind and it makes you less anxious. It also helps if you are a shallow breather; take some deep breaths, and continue this with your counting. Let's say you count from 1-10; slowly take a deep breath on the five, repeat it, and then take two deep breaths. Continue doing this as long as necessary and eventually your anxiety will fade away.

The only limit is in your head! Trying to get over your anxiety isn't easy, it's not a rush job, even though those suffering from anxiety would like it to be. Although it's painful to begin with, there are little things you can do to help yourself. As well as looking at your symptoms, you can look at the physical environment that you have — what things do you add to it regularly? It could be fresh flowers, new towels, curtains, or bedspreads. These are little things, but they affect your living environment and how you live within it.

And, are you allowing your life to get too cluttered? Do you hoard paperwork, furniture, clothing, or food? If you do, it's time to let go of some of these things in your life. Clearing out the clutter will give your mind more clarity, enabling you to work on existing projects, instead of being continuously worried about past ones.

Another key element, as I have already implied, is cleanliness: cleaning is essential to your wellbeing. Your surrounding should reflect on yourself and your hygiene levels. It should be a place you can welcome people into. Though, if you cannot, then there is an immediate problem and this highlights the soul aspect of your life.

It's often difficult letting people into your private space. So, when you are caught out, it's only you that is to blame if you have left your bin unemptied or, for example, if you have not cleaned the bath. These are all things that you should be doing routinely. It should be as regular as clockwork. Especially if you live on your own, as there is no excuse because you are the only one accountable for your own living conditions. And there is always something that can be tweaked for the better.

Now, think of yourself like your house or apartment. What are your daily needs? Let's start with breakfast. This should be on the essential list. Do not go anywhere without it, or make plans to have it as you leave the house.

Social interaction is a must-have in your daily routine. You need to ask a few questions here:
- How do you plan on getting it?
- What efforts are you making yourself?
- Do you look presentable enough?
- Is your manner playful and approachable?
- Is your demeanour akin to the dark destroyer, making people want to avoid you altogether?

Answer these questions honestly and get to work —

it makes all the difference. And of course, cleanliness is not essential for being sociable but, in the end, it's better to be sociable and clean.

So, take steps to make your appearance more presentable, just like you would do to your home. I am sure you'd love doing a home improvement project, but that's not immediately conceivable, whereas buying new clothes is. But it is worth budgeting for both scenarios. Remember — your home is your sanctuary from the world outside, just as your body is a statement of your health and your intentions.

Now, what else is important for yourself daily?

Some mental exercises can never go wrong — private research or a hobby could help give your nerves a run for their money. It's the biggest goal for you to find out what makes you tick and what gives you instant fulfilment. This is not related to illicit drugs, or alcohol consumption, or even overeating.

Now, let's ask some difficult questions, beginning with one of the easier ones — what gets you out of bed in the mornings? Is it a belief system? Is it a job? A partner? A child? What is it exactly that gets you out of the bed every morning and ready for the challenges of the day? For some people, animals are the answer. For many of us living on our own, we are all we have to get up for.

Once you have your answer, you have worked out the easy part. They do say to start at the very beginning of these things. If it is a belief system, it is likely to be a positive one, even if you get out of bed to make yourself a cup of coffee and you believe that you can now start your day — it's a positive sign.

The first thing I do in the mornings is feed my cat. I always have enough food for her. I wish I were that diligent with my own nutritional needs. Next, I go into the bathroom to get cleaned up, but then I usually put on any clothes that I can find from the closet. I do not make an effort to have them set out neatly for the day, which is a mistake because I always have time beforehand to prepare clothes.

I have very few distractions in my life. I do not even have a TV to engross me for hours, so it's just social media pages that I enthusiastically use daily. However, they do not take up too much of my time.

So, I do have the time to do things. I have the intention to get up in the mornings, even if it's only to make sure that my cat is fed on time. But what am I doing with my time? I have so much of it now and, more importantly, what *could* I be doing with it? What do I want to get out of my day? Is it just to show up or to be an active participator? If it's the latter, then there are certain ground rules.

Have you had your breakfast? Are you clean? Did you sleep well last night? If not, then why not? What are you going to do about not sleeping properly? Do you need to take a bath before bed? Do you need to exercise more? What are you showing up for, and is your contribution being noted? Do you get fulfilment from where you are right now? How is appreciation shown? If you are going somewhere where you are getting no fulfilment, have you asked yourself the question: why are you still going there? What makes you stand up and be counted? What fires and motivates you?

These are the things that should never leave you, you should never give up. If it's a passion for cinema that you have, then follow it — visit the theatre or maybe head over to the cinema to catch the next summer blockbuster. There is always a new slant on seeing things from every generation, and sometimes you have not seen it the first time around.

The world is your oyster! One thing that we do not often ask in these situations is: what do I *truly* need?

Yes, we could all count on friends to help us more in our life, or even acquaintances, to help us do things. I spoke to a therapist years ago, and after our conversation, she said to me, "We are human beings, not human doings."

I remember another one saying, "Don't write lists. Lists are your problems in life. You write too many lists." The funny thing is that I actually listened to her advice and realized that it was the most damaging thing I could have done. As soon as I didn't have a list to complete, it was as if I had no reason to exist — there seemed nothing to do anymore. In fact, for many years, I lay in the quagmire, actually believing and taking comfort in the thought that there was nothing left to do anymore. I couldn't have been more wrong or more wrongly advised.

So, for many years, I just drifted aimlessly into anything and everything remotely interesting. Then gradually, I lost interest, not seeing the point of anything — without being nihilistic. There were points where it was a mutually satisfying time, but without any guidance, I wasn't able to benefit from it.

It gets more challenging when you are older — people

are not as willing to help on account of you not being a novice, and based on, "Why should I help you?" You may have to work out a lot of things yourself, which may require hard work and grit on your part. It is a relentless and continuous process and when you have achieved something, there is always the next thing to accomplish or move on to.

Well, that's how it should be!

I've managed to do just that, or let's just say that I have acquired that level in life. Wow! It feels so nice to say that I am on the next level, or should be upgraded to one at least. Saying all this helps — consolatory thoughts help. Everything might not be as readily available to you as it was when you were younger, but as soon as you set your mind to change, you will be amazed how much help is out there, just waiting for you!

You have to look for help in places accessible to you — be it traditional or non-traditional. Ask around, ask friends and acquaintances, and it helps if you know what you're asking for. Knowing what kind of help you need saves you and other peoples' time, too.

Always have a plan of action — know what you want help with. How much time it's going to take. Know your commitment levels and how others function. It's best not to do these things half-heartedly. As I said, it takes you to the next level, and if you are always striving for the next level, you are constantly moving forward. This is the momentum you need to simply keep going. It's another thing worth getting up for in the morning, just knowing that you are going to be busy in completing something. Knowing that there is a plan for you and that you are an active part of it — knowing that you are the master of your destiny, and every day you are working towards a project, and a completion. This is an ideal drive for the day, something to put in your diary, an obvious talking point, something that will enable you to interact.

CHAPTER 4 — THE HEALING JOURNEY

Success is the ability to go from failure to failure without losing your enthusiasm.

– Ayn Rand

Taking things forward from here and following these techniques to heal the emotional paralysis is a good idea. You need to know your likes and dislikes — something that moves and motivates you. Otherwise, you would never be fully invested in something. When you have too much time on your hands, what is your motivation to reach beyond yourself out into space? When all you can think is, I do not know what to do. This is a self-limiting belief. It stems actually from abundance, a place where there is so much choice — you are overwhelmed by freedom of choice!

Thinking and saying that you do not know what to do might indicate that you are going through some sort of depression — or maybe not. Sometimes, it's truly difficult to reach a decision. Sometimes this is out of fear, fear of making the wrong decision, and being left high and dry at a critical moment. But let me tell you, this is the wrong mindset to establish right off the bat. When you come from a place of abundance, you are free to choose and make informed decisions. Your happiness hinges on it and that is all that should matter.

The dread that you have in you about making the wrong decisions, is what stops you from trying in the first place — it's the fear of failure. When you get into a situation like this, an idea to help you make a decision is to find out what value would be added to your existence and the situation if you take a certain step or move in a certain direction. Make sure you love the reasons for it. What purpose does this decision fulfil in your life? Is it the only decision that you have? Why do you feel that you have to make it now? What are you putting off by not making decisions in your life?

Once you have made your decision, make sure that you are happy with it. There is no point taking the time to make it just to be unsure or discontent with it afterwards. But be reassured, decisions are not set in stone, and they do not have to be permanent.

Everything is changeable and that is the best way to look at it... There is always an opt-out option, but it's important to make the decision first. Show a level of commitment that means you are operating at a functional level. The worry always when you make a decision is, can you go back on it? But taking the time to make the right decision means that you shouldn't have to worry so much. That being said, you will have much more clarity now. Just make sure that decisions are always a part of the overall plan you have for your life. It saves you from making the wrong moves.

Once you have started your way into a more organized life, there will be no stopping you. It's easier to make more decisions on those lines now that you have already made one. And there! You have immediately reduced your fear of organizing yourself and getting things done. The proficiency with which you can eradicate your fears is how you become less anxious in the first place. Make well-informed decisions. Reduce the risk of anxiety by telling yourself that you are in control over your life. There isn't anything to worry about. Everything will work out fine as long as you have taken the necessary steps in the first place. There is no need to be anxious.

Anxiety itself is something that demands to heal. Whether it is healing from deep emotional trauma or healing from something physically traumatic, it heals in stages. As is the case, many types of deep emotional trauma require healing. They could be anything — for instance, losing a loved one, severe bullying, being attacked or abused in some way. In the end, one has to learn — as hard as it sounds — that it is possible to recover from it. This is an essential part of learning that has to take place. It is the most difficult thing to come to terms with, but essentially if we do not get over it, we cannot or will not move on from where we are standing right now, emotionally. It is the hardest lesson that we have to learn, however learning it, and learning it well, will be the key to our success.

For example, a traumatic experience like losing a loved one shakes a person on so many levels. The grieving process is something that can take as long as a whole lifetime or just a handful of years — it varies for every person. Losing someone close to us — whether it is a best friend, a family member, or a partner — is bound to change our outlook on life. It changes our perspective and allows us to value people. Being used to having that person around, and then all of a sudden, having them removed from your life permanently is guaranteed to leave a big void in your life. That void fills up in its own time; you have little control over it. You will always be looking back in a state of pain and regret if you have not been able to gain closure.

It is, by far, the hardest thing you have to move on from in your life, emotionally. You are in a state where your life has literally been turned upside down and inside out. But it is okay to feel that way — you might feel overwhelmed at times, or emotionally struggling and looking for a shoulder to cry on — it's just part of understanding your grief. You feel that your grief is now a burden, and everyone has heard the story before. You have heard the phrase "get over it" so many times and you just cannot do it. You are left with a void that needs to be filled.

They say time is a great healer, but if you are at the beginning of your journey, that's not very comforting. When you feel that you do not know what to do anymore, your reason for living might also have changed now that the significant other is no longer in your life. How do you heal from this sort of trauma?

Healing comes in layers, and at first, you will need the support of your friends and family. It's hard to say, but at this time in your life, sometimes friends are not around — they are married off or maybe have relocated far away — so this step can even feel harder for you. But many people have gone through it before you and several will discover the meaning of grief later on.

You can always reach out to organizations that support people in their time of difficulties like the Samaritans and Cruise. You can also visit a counsellor if things get really bad, and discuss your feelings with them.

Grief is like being alone again. It is the worst kind of loneliness there is and sadly, you have to learn to go through it on your own. It's not an experience that can be shared as such. You have to find your method of coping with the effects of bereavement. As I said, this takes a bit of time. The good news is eventually, with the right sort of support, you can get over the most painful of feelings. That isn't to say that you won't revisit these feelings of emptiness and sadness from time to time. It is natural that when you reflect on your life, you are bound to feel the pangs of injustice, but it's alright. Things eventually get better — trust me, they do. You learn to live with it, and that's when the healing begins. You have to continue to go through the same emotional experiences so that you can rework your new level of healing. Once you have reached this, it can only make you stronger and better equipped to deal with any future life events.

So, the healing journey begins. However, if left unchecked, this is a stumbling block that leads to anxiety. Any hidden grief is bound to surface eventually and it can occur most unpleasantly, emerging in a range of personal problems. It is so important to spend time talking about grief with someone, preferably a professional, as grief affects people differently and professional counsellors are equipped to handle this pain.

I will put myself in the spotlight. When I was 15 years old, as I was about to take my exams and having just reached puberty, my father suddenly died of a heart attack. I came home one day and he just wasn't there anymore.

My mother immediately began grieving, whereas I didn't mention it to anyone. I was very embarrassed about my situation and I felt like I shouldn't tell anyone about my dad's untimely demise. I mistakenly felt that the burden would be too much for them and I didn't want them to feel sorry for me. So, when people mentioned him, I spoke as if he was still alive, so no one would ask me any questions, but 15 years later, I had a breakdown and that was something I had to deal with alone.

For 15 years, I didn't grieve. Even to this day, I have not grieved properly or addressed the problems with a counsellor — it is something that I still need to do as I have not had full closure. For me, this is an open wound. To this day, I cannot talk about my feelings around death. I immediately find it so uncomfortable that I start flip-flopping around the subject, steering it away from that unwanted conversation. The trauma I went through was so painful that I am still unwilling to discuss it with anyone on a deeper level. But I realized that this was inhibiting the therapeutic process and leaving me in a constant state of angst. I kept thinking, maybe I should try meditating on this issue because it's not going away. I reasoned that the sooner I dealt with it, the better. This would also resolve my other traumas related to feelings of abandonment in childhood.

When we no longer know what to do, we have to come to our real work, and when we no longer know what way to go, we have begun our real journey.

— Wendell Barry

So, it is the new times in our lives that we need to explore. These are the times where we evaluate our existence, give ourselves a life inventory, and think about what we have gained so far. What have we left to achieve? And how likely it is that we will achieve anything more than what we have achieved so far? It's an assessment of our life goals. What were the good parts? What was it that stopped us from succeeding? What were the circumstances in our lives that made for the detours taking us off our natural path? And did we come back to our path by any route?

The real work is when we spend hours debating with ourselves over the fact of whether we are choosing the right things for our lives: have we met our expectations? What are our expectations now for our lives? And how have we ranked them? Have we set our sights too low? Or are they way beyond our limitations? Are they unrealistic?

The real work helps fathom these things out, but you'd be foolish to think that this part is the easy part — it isn't — that is why we say the real work begins here.

Sometimes, what is necessary is real investigative work — looking at your personality from all angles — looking at aspects such as your self-worth and evaluating the status of your self-esteem. Does it come from your occupation? Or does it come from your status? Or perhaps you have a skill that is exceptional that not many people have? Finding those things out helps bring the focus back to you and your needs. To maintain healthy self-esteem, you have to know the core things that help build esteem in the first place. Once you have outlined what they are, it's time to nourish them and maintain them as well. There will be times when days will not go according to plan — days when everything will go wrong — your self-worth and self-esteem will take a hit during those times. You need to practise self-love and self-care to keep yourself intact.

You are protecting yourself from the onslaught of negative thought patterns and have nourished your spirit sufficiently so that you can take on whatever comes next without the added fear that you would normally take on-board otherwise. Your approach to fear itself would be different. In fact, it has been said that a certain amount of fear is healthy and if you do something you fear every day, your ability to conquer it gets easier.

For example, if, like me, you have a fear of heights, you might think you will never be able to do a parachute jump. Still, you could manage to go on a ski lift or abseil down a building. These are two things that I have achieved by my willingness to try and conquer a long-standing fear. I had a fear of heights for most of my adult life, and I faced it.

But there are other fears that you can learn to combat in the same way. They may be associated with social skills. One of the most common fears is being in a room with many unknown people, not knowing how or when to start a conversation. It seems that as much as you fear this situation, the more you do it, the easier it becomes. So, putting yourself into situations that challenge you is a way to meet your fear head-on, and in this circumstance, you might have to ask yourself the question — what is the worst thing that could happen?

In my days working in management, I was asked to be a speaker and to talk about the scheme that I was promoting, so I decided I needed to get help from some expert trainers and enrolled in a series of courses.

It was at this time that I was asked to address a wider audience. With the training that I previously had, I was confident enough to be able to do it.

But this isn't the case with everybody. Once, I was attending a welcoming party and they had a guy speak in front of a large audience. This guy was extremely nervous — to the extent that while speaking and taking a glass of water, he broke the glass and the water went everywhere. He wasn't able to calm his nerves after that and his speech went from bad to worse. He was *that* anxious about a speech. Coupled with a large audience, the pressure was too much for him to take...

It was very difficult to watch him, but the audience wasn't particularly sympathetic. So, he left feeling very nervous and doubtful that he would want to undertake anything like that again. Both of these levels of anxiety were unnecessary.

He had a fear of public speaking, but he might be much better at small talk, which other people fear instead. It seemed such a shame, as I saw the whole room witness his public meltdown, because it was so unnecessary. If he had counted to ten and just slowed down a little, he would have seen that everyone was interested in what he had to say. And he could have left out the bits he was unprepared for. That being said, maybe I wouldn't have taken on the responsibility of covering for someone at such short notice, not completely knowing the subject, when it was an important presentation.

But he did admonish himself in front of everyone, which made matters worse for him. Later on, he became a nervous wreck and had a full meltdown, as I mentioned before. This is the power of negative self-talk; it brings out the fear in you and magnifies it, so you're no longer trying to get over a molehill, but a fully formed mountain that's ready to crush you under its weight.

It is always good to be mindful of that inner critic. When it starts its rumblings and ramblings, if it's leading you more and more into discomfort, you need to suppress that trigger as it will lead to more fear-ridden anxiety and nervousness.

So, your *real* journey starts here. Learn to tackle your fears and do not forget to love yourself. It is the only way to begin your journey out of a fear-ridden life. If you are trying your best, you do not need to put yourself down. By doubting yourself, you are not helping the situation. All it does is increase your level of fear and destroys your self-worth, or what's left of it.

Being burdened with doubts does not serve anyone, least of all yourself. This adds to the negative thought patterns and becomes a part of them. It can immobilize you when you have thought something through and finally mustered the courage to do it. A lingering doubt does not just make you feel uncomfortable, it also makes you question some of your core beliefs.

You might backtrack if you are unsure of yourself and the direction you should take but, again, it does not help anyone. The more confident you are, the better you can go about your day and the changes you wish to make to it. Any self-deprecating thought is a big No.

Therefore, out of all the negative self-talk and inner

critique, doubting is by far the worst enemy of your soul, as it undermines your self-confidence the most. This undermining behaviour stops you from moving forward and can have debilitating effects on your wellbeing, too. The best way to confront a doubting mind is to remove insecurities, of every shape and form, that impede your progress.

There are often thought-patterns telling you that you are not going to be as good as your peers, or maybe that you are just not good enough for anything. This type of thinking can stem from a lack of self-worth during the early years — it could be due to a lack of acknowledgment as a child, having been overlooked or not receiving enough praise. When you are ignored and sidestepped often, it's hard to build up a level of self-confidence on your own. You need to get some outward approval and when this does not come around often, it's easy to feel deflated or unhappy with yourself.

It is at this moment that you need to find your inner resolve and work towards total self-acceptance.

CHAPTER 5 — SELF-ESTEEM

Spread love everywhere you go. Let no one ever come to you without feeling happier.

– Henry Ford

We get to know about our self-worth from our achievements in life. But if we have not achieved anything, we do not have a yardstick with which we can measure our worth — many of us are stuck in this rut. I had a period of my life when I was unemployed. Previously, I had managed to gain my self-worth by achieving a certain level at work, completing certain key projects well, and building a status with regards to my position. At that time, I was confident in my abilities and worked the hours necessary to achieve my goals.

However, I worked more than the hours required of me and I had a very limited social life. My levels of self-esteem correlated with the quantity and quality of my work, and any socializing I did was in work, causing work to consume my life.

Subsequently, I had a mental breakdown because of the long hours and the constant focus on work. But of course, I couldn't see it coming at the time.

There is an example of all worth being misplaced that is derived only from a job. Once the job disappears, so does the self-worth. This is why you have to find something better than a job to create your self-worth — something that can withstand the storm and something that you have with you at all times. It does not matter if you lose your job, you still have this self-worth.

How do you attract this sort of self-worth with

renewed self-esteem? Firstly, you have to think positively about yourself. You have to invest time in your happiness. Secondly, by doing things that you love regularly, like going to the cinema, sailing, archery, taking that dance class, going to a yoga class, or enrolling in an art class.

Take up a new hobby. It does not matter what it is, as long as you are engaged.

There are a lot of things that can help with self-worth at this level. As well as boosting you up, you simply need to channel your energies forward for a change — so that you're not stuck in the quagmire of angst and indecision. All these actions are putting you in the best place to move forward.

Say, you have the desire to attract new friends in your life, you can do this by attending classes and meeting people, so that's two birds with one stone. Generally, that's the best way to think of things. What could I be doing now to help me with my private goals? Despite not having certain things in your life like a job, a partner, children or a large amount of disposable income that people consider essential, how else do you think you can find happiness? There is always a way.

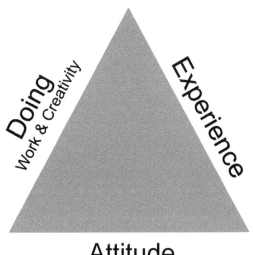

Viktor Frankl's (1964) **Meaning Triangle**

Doing: work & creativity
Giving something to the world through self-expression, such as; work, good deeds, art, music, writing, invention.

Experience
Receiving from the world through nature, culture, relationships, interactions with others and our environment, spirituality.

Attitude
Even if we can't change our situation or circumstance, we can still choose our attitude toward a situation, condition or suffering — changing the way we think about life situations, seeing a different perspective, and

simply looking at it a different way.

Frankl found that even in extreme suffering, we can change the way we think about a situation, to give us a sense of purpose. Our purpose affects our self-esteem because when we have clear understanding of our purpose, we feel better about ourselves and our future. The Meaning Triangle helps us identify our purpose by breaking down where we find true meaning in our lives, finding out what we are drawn to, what we value and what we would do more of given the opportunity. (Source: getselfhelp.co.uk)

One way of looking at life is by looking at the 'large amount of money at your disposal' scenario. What would you do differently if you had a large disposable income? And what things would stay the same? How would this affect your purpose? If we are talking about me, I would travel more if I had a large disposable income — I would travel far and wide and journal my travelling pictorially with anecdotes. I wouldn't waste my time worrying about what clothes I should wear as I do now.

I would just get rid of at least 80% of my clothes and buy exactly what I need for a change in the shop, there and then. I would not waste time searching the internet for bargain deals that look markedly different than what is shown.

Being worried about your look can be linked to your disposable income and how confident you feel in your clothes. It is preferable to avoid just making do with your clothes and instead, separating them into weekday and weekend wear — separate the day clothes, nightclothes, going out clothes and gym clothes. These also reflect part of your personality and the more time you spend organizing this part of your life, the happier you will be, as this is *your* persona going out into the world. It says — I am ready to meet any new challenges. I am prepared to clean and become organized. I have taken the first steps to improve my wellbeing.

Make sure that the way you appear to the outside world is your best, with whatever means you have. Display the persona you want to have, in the clothes that define your new style.

For a short period of my life, I travelled around with a homeless man, and as time went on, he became aware of the state of his own attire more and more. Although much of it was donations, he still wanted to give an outward impression that he was looking after himself, and he sought out clothes that were appealing to him. He didn't just wear anything. So, if a man with no roof over his head can organize himself and appear decent, what excuse does someone who has more than a roof over their head have?

It is this desire — to want something more than what is being offered to you, a purpose — that helps you achieve your dreams. This homeless man in question managed to secure himself a home eventually, but it had a lot to do with his outward appearance. It is important to be conscious of your outward appearance; it affects what is being attracted to you. Making that effort to appear clean and tidy means that you have put thought into your appearance. You should be going above and beyond to physically establish your personality. It is a good start to the day and can only end on a high.

Putting the wheels in motion at the beginning of the day is another way to raise your self-esteem — having people comment on how you look, and how well presented you are can mean a lot. It shows that you have put the effort in already. You are ready to start the day, and by starting it on the right foot, you are more likely to have a productive day, and of course, your appearance will be noted and appreciated. There goes that well-dressed individual, they must really take good care of their life.

If I have a problem or an issue with something, I'm more likely to go to this person for advice and help, rather than someone who is unkempt and does not look like they want to participate in life.

Someone who takes pride in their appearance takes pride in other aspects of their life, too. They possibly have got their home life sorted, and they have nailed the getting breakfast element, as well as the rest of the meals they need to stay healthy. They probably have a fitness regime in place too. They either go to the gym or do regular steps to meet their daily requirement in order to stay healthy.

So, appearance says a lot about a person and how they appear ready for the challenges of the day. It's very much like putting on your armour, or the armour of the Lord, to go out with strength, knowing that you are prepared for all eventualities. Clothe yourself with humility as well as an attitude for the task at hand. Rid yourself of all anxiety and fear by anticipating good things, because you have started on a good foot, you have made an effort to look at your outward appearance, and you have credited yourself for being worthy first.

Give yourself the chance of a good day by awakening to thoughts of your needs. Expect good things when you put in the effort to make your day better. It's easy to just curl up in a ball and sleep off all the problems that you have, but eventually, when you wake up, if you have not dealt with those problems, they are still going to exist and they will be hanging around your neck like a heavy gold chain.

When you show up for the day, make sure that you are not too tired, but instead refreshed. Make sure that you have the necessary amount of nutrients in your body so that you can function, because without rest and nutrients the body won't work at all — it refuses to function properly. All you get is a sluggish response and a half-hearted stab at life because you are not ready for the day. You have not put on your armour of the Lord. You have not said any of the affirmations that take you away from feeling useless and incomplete.

You are not showing up to work things out if you are just about dragging yourself up in the mornings. That means you have forgotten to think about yourself first. This is something that you have to understand and accept; you are the master of your destiny — the captain of your ship. Anywhere you go, it's because you have led yourself there, so do not blame anyone else, or praise anyone else, for your choices in life.

You are the one in control, it's just about where you want to go next in life, and this should be the most exciting and challenging aspect of living. This implies that you are not just showing up anymore, you are actively participating in your own life. This is *your* life!

What do you want to do with it? There are huge opportunities once you realize that you are in control.

You have taken charge, and you are now in the driving seat!

One thing that you need to get rid of in your life is the many lies that have kept you where you are today.

These are the lies that your ego has told you. The lies that some friends and some family members may have told you. The lies that you have been telling yourself for years and ended up believing.

Today is the time to start — what about the lie that said you weren't good enough to start writing a book? As someone that has never found it difficult to write before, goodness, I found it difficult to cope with the writer's block that I'd get writing this book. Although I have never been a writer of stories, I am generally a writer of letters; I was always able to express myself with the written word. If I had a problem, I could just write it out.

If I was thinking of something in the future, I could plan things by forecasting, using vision boards, the works. So, these things prove that I can write even though I thought that I couldn't. This confirms that it's a lie that I cannot write, I obviously can, and it's important to discover this kind of truth about yourself.

Besides this, another lie that I tell myself is that I do not have any friends. The truth is that I do have friends, but they are not necessarily there for me all the time, or at the times that I need them to be there. This is a realization in life, and it shows me that I have not always been around for my friends when they needed me either.

It's a lie to say that I have made myself readily available to my friends all the time, when I have not. So, what you expect from them is sometimes more than you deserve. If you think of the biblical quote, "do unto others that which you would have done to yourself." (Matthew 7:12) You can see clearly that the lies you have been saying — for example, that you are always available to them when you weren't — dictates the sort of relationship you have with them.

The same applies for family, though it is more likely that some lies are left hidden in families. There might be sibling rivalry because one sibling gets all the attention. But this can be masked by a series of lies, indicating that they get on perfectly fine, when in truth, they do not. Instead, one always seems to get away with things, whereas the other seems to have to fulfil a set of tasks on a daily or weekly basis. One could be held in higher regard than the other because of an achieved status or a dominant characteristic which has been nurtured through their childhood.

The perpetual lies, that insinuate that everything is hunky-dory, are pretty routine at family get-togethers and reunions. This can be quite painful — having to endure an event and still trying to put a lid on things — to avoid conflict and arguments. It seems that in families there are complications because of the history of their home lives. It seems to be recorded in each individual's brain and replayed sporadically, giving a different angle to the same events each time.

Gatherings can be dreadful, as you are constantly trying not to step on anyone's toes. But you still try to impress family members with whatever activity or role you are assigned. This is the stage where they expect something from you each time you come to the table. But sometimes, the expectations can be too high for you — which is why the tendency to avoid such gatherings exists.

Their lies would have you believe that they do not judge you heavily, because you are a relative, but they do. The interrogation you have within a family setting is supposed to prepare you for the outside world, so it should really be a safe environment for you to learn and grow.

It is in this environment that we learn our fundamental life lessons. We learn to make our mistakes and have them corrected for us. We learn to define our boundaries and become an individual in our own right.

Another lie we might tell ourselves is that we are good with money. We can handle our affairs without help — this is something only a few people can handle.

I was in a situation where I had quite a substantial debt, but I was in denial over it. When the bills came through the door, I did nothing, and even posted them back to the people I was in debt to. All I was doing was making things worse. The debts were eventually forwarded to a debt collection organization, forcing me to take immediate action. I had nothing to hide behind anymore. I gradually agreed on a payment plan which suited both the debt collectors and me, and eventually we worked it out amicably — at least I don't have to pay interest anymore. But for so long, I was living under this lie that everything was going to be fine. I was thinking this while I could barely afford to eat, and the rest of the bills were piling up.

I had gone on a spending spree and was readily

buying clothes that I could hardly afford, and that was — in all intentions — inappropriate. I became a hoarder of clothes, most of which I later gave away to charity. What a waste of money. And the thing is, it took me years to realize this was unnatural behaviour. I had to knock this off my list. It wasn't serving me and was causing me to go into debt, so I decided to curtail my expenditure. Everything I did not need in my life, I got rid of straight away. Now, I am only living on the bare essentials that I truly need.

I was still able to save some money, miraculously, and this is something I continue to do even today. Putting money away for a rainy day. And it curtails to the lie that I'm not preparing for my future. Every penny I save towards my future is an investment in myself.

It gives me a sense of security to know that there is a fund set up, waiting for me, if all other avenues are closed. Living a frugal life is the best way to understand money and not waste it. Recognizing the value of money and the benefits of having it when you need it helps to ease the levels of anxiety that you have. By being careful with your purchases, and only buying what you need, you soon realize what it is that you actually need. Saving for the wants in life makes you question how badly you want something because there is often a sacrifice involved, especially when money is in inconsistent supply.

Making your money work for you is important. You should be able to go away on a holiday if you direly need to because nothing is worse than staring at the same walls from winter to summer, especially when you are going through a rough patch.

Do what I do — set aside some money for travel expenses, because its good to broaden your horizon whenever you get a chance. It could be a weekend getaway or a week off in the Cotswolds. Whatever it is, it is a well-deserved break that gives you some fresh air, a change of scenery, and should leave you feeling revitalized.

Planning money for these things is, therefore, vital. What it really does is lower your levels of anxiety — anxiety often comes with the feeling of being stuck in a rut, doing the same thing day in and day out, without having the freedom to explore anything beyond the usual four walls, being closed in mind and space, not getting a chance to appreciate nature or your living environment.

And not being conscious of your surroundings affects your mental health as well.

With anxiety, it is often the case that we accept our environment for what it is — even if it is cluttered and messy — thus affecting the energy around us. It is in this state that we accept things without necessarily having a willingness to change them. To our disadvantage, we often stay in stagnated environments where there isn't enough flow of energy surrounding us. This is the first thing that we need to do something about!

Let's say, even if you are just having breakfast in these environments, and the nature of anxiety is such that it is receptive to new things — or in fact, desires new things and new experiences — it is important to counter this anxiety with the knowledge that you can change your environment, as it really helps to alleviate it.

There is nothing worse than stagnating your schedule to feed your anxious thoughts. It only magnifies the problem at hand. It also stays and grows more as you do nothing about the situation. If you are scared to step in and rule over the situation, sooner or later, anxiety will kick in again. The less movement there is, the more entrapped you will feel, and the more caged-in you feel, the lesser the likelihood of you reaching out beyond the confines of the quagmire.

Beyond the room of despair is where you will find the real help, and it is you who will decide how exactly to get there and get it. You have to be cautious at this stage and move away from your despondency carefully.

Whilst it is relatively easy to get yourself out of certain situations, an issue like this, which is deeply entrenched, needs a miracle. That's what you will be asking for, whether you pray about it directly or follow careful guidelines to get yourself out of the mess you find yourself in. But where you are now is a no-go area, where no one wants to help you. You have brought it on yourself with fearful thinking and inaction.

What are these guidelines? How do you get out of it? This is going to be your most difficult task yet. But if you can pull yourself through this, you will likely be able to pull yourself through anything.

So, what do you have to do first? The first thing you have to do is to remove yourself physically from your state of stagnation. Whether it is a dead-end job, that habit of staying inside for most of the day, getting up late, not feeding yourself properly, or some other thing. Firstly, identify the unhelpful pattern in your life and attack it aggressively. It's the only way to confront this kind of passivity.

You have identified it as being bad for you. Congratulations! Now it's time to do something about it. Break the chains that shackle you, and hold you back. Attack them from every angle. If you are leaving the house late at night and sleeping in the next day, then set an early alarm for the next few mornings to get yourself back to your regular waking time. Start buying yourself nutritional food, and do not avoid breakfast. I cannot stress this enough: make sure that you have breakfast in the mornings.

CHAPTER 6 — BAD HABITS

What lies behind us and what lies before us are tiny matters compared to what lies within us.
— Oliver Wendell Holmes

Here's the thing — fear only shows up when you stop showing up for your life and commitments. When that happens, everything falls apart. You forget your priorities. These are the things that organize your days and weeks. These are the things that fill your months to come. It is important to show up and participate in life, otherwise your life becomes derelict, while others move on with theirs. You cannot move forward because you have not made a plan, or the plan you have made hasn't been executed.

Fearful thinking occurs when you realize that you have done nothing substantial in your life, and there isn't anything in the pipeline. Fear destroys confidence in every way.

So, we can establish that fear comes from inactivity. We know what we can do to remove fear in our lives. Fear comes from states where you do not know what you are doing but have no intention of doing anything about it. In other cases, you may have an intention to do something, but you still do not do anything about it.

It is a place where time loses meaning, and it eventually catches up with you when you find that you have done nothing in its place. It is this state of nothingness that needs to be addressed and fast, before more time goes by and nothing is done. Wasted time that does not help anyone is called empty time, meaning the sort of time that when asked what have you been doing with your life, you cannot quantify it because it's just unaccountable time.

The aim is to be responsible for your time, so you have an inventory of time spent and you can tell these stories of how you have spent your time. You should not be caught in the vacuous expanse that might involve sleeping too long, running too many errands, not taking enough time out for yourself to do the things you enjoy doing. Losing memories of the things you like doing is dangerous and not right.

You must try to remember, despite the anxiety, the things that make you feel less anxious and the things that make you more excited. These things will propel you forwards, and you can do these things no matter what circumstances you find yourself in. If you are having a bad day, it's good to bear in mind what you can do to keep going and maintain a positive mood. Make an effort to know what these things are and where they occur in your life. It is so important to have these things close to you at your disposal, especially when you have a series of bad days, it is the best way of lifting your spirits.

So, use these memories constantly. The things that make you feel brighter and more energetic are the ones you should be focusing on. I assure you, you will find your road to inner peace.

A huge problem for people suffering from anxiety is loneliness. Loneliness can manifest itself in many ways. But whatever way it comes up, it is destructive. Feeling lonely happens to everyone at some time in their life; some experience periods of loneliness, others feel isolated for the most part. However, feeling lonely, all or most of the time is not great for our anxiety levels. And it can occur obviously because of comparison with other people and their lifestyles. This could be especially due to what we see on social media with all our virtual friends' and people's posts. It establishes meeting up physically as a necessary social interaction, and the pressure for someone experiencing loneliness to meet people is enormous.

It would be easier if they kept to their usual circles, but they can feel left out easily. For example, if their social media feeds are not being picked up — if they have stopped going out and socializing, or find it hard to be in social groups because of social anxiety, they will start ostracising themselves. This compounds their problem, and they fail to reach out to people for help of any sort. Social interaction is essential for good mental health, so if you notice that someone is secluded, it's good to invite them out. This way, they can come out of themselves.

The worst thing is when it develops into a habit, it becomes very hard to break. It is possible, though, to break the habits that are built on the basis of loneliness. By encouraging the individual to come out more — to spend less time by themselves and to be part of a group or group activities — you could help them immensely. This is one way of shaking the blanket of loneliness off of individuals and helping them move forwards in an interactive way. I found out that I usually feel lonely first thing in the morning. When I initially wake up and am deciding what to do with my day is when I feel I am at my worst.

But then, by the time evening has come along, I will have done something to be out of the house, and end up feeling less conscious of my surroundings and environment. Ideally, I should write down the night before what I'm doing the next day in order to prevent some of the anxiety I usually experience in the mornings. Loneliness is, therefore, something that affects me intermittingly. It does not always have to be in the mornings that I feel lonely, it can be in the afternoon and the evening, too.

I counter this sinking feeling by being busy. There are so many things you can do to keep busy — this varies for everyone. For me, cleaning is one of them, and it always needs to be done. Cleaning your environment is one way of feeling less lonely, especially if you get into it. It can distract you for hours, and at the end of it, it always makes you feel better mentally. Getting rid of the clutter builds on that feeling.

Things like keeping busy at work, taking on a voluntary position, offering to help at your local Church, being more active in your local community — all of these things can help you to feel less lonely and more involved in the things going on around you.

My struggle with anxiety started some time ago. Before that, I had experienced bouts of depression and psychosis for which I had been hospitalized, but there was one year that my psychosis had become so bad that I didn't realize how ill I was. I had been trying to function as much as I could by doing daily tasks, such as; preparing food for lunch, going on courses, and completing various assignments. However, I hadn't been taking my medication for months, and my mental health was going from bad to worse.

I found it hard to communicate with people, and I had some problems that I felt I was not comfortable discussing with anyone. That situation worsened, and I ended up being trapped in my bubble, experiencing life as a loner, and hardly engaging with people. When I did engage with them, I found it difficult to have a sustained and meaningful relationship.

My anxiety got so bad that it affected my breathing at night. Sometimes I felt I was suffocating and had to sleep with the window wide open. I went to the Doctors to see if there were any other underlying causes, but she confirmed it was anxiety. This is how frightening anxiety can be.

This, I believe, all stemmed from a need to interact with people, but having social anxiety meant that I was not equipped with the necessary skills to engage with people normally. This social anxiety got worse, and I found that when I went out, I spoke less and less to people, and was always conscious of my failures all the time. I would only ever remark on how many times I had been ill. This would stop me straight away in a conversation as I had tried to disguise depressive episodes to such an extent that they seeped out in other ways. The more I tried to deny my depression or anxiety, the more the problem manifested.

This shame I've felt about my illness has come about because of the stigma associated with this type of mental illness. My family also had a different approach when dealing with it, and that was by not acknowledging it. Rather than dwelling on it, they wanted me to come out of it as soon as possible. I'm different now from how I was before. I used to be a lot quieter and was incapable of breaking out of it in the moment. I was always self-conscious about my actions — what I was doing and saying — and this living in fear had taken over my life when anxiety came to visit. It came to the point when I was choosing food, I felt fear about getting it organized.

There are so many ways that fear presents itself in my life. It is mostly trying to do things differently than before. Things that would have almost certainly aided my recovery, it seems.

Even though I had taken to reading many self-help books before writing this book, I thought it was essential to be authentic and say how dark and long the struggle can be. Being truthful, with others and myself, constantly reminds me of how far I have come. But it also outlines my struggles to you, so you can see that dealing with anxiety and depression is a real process.

So, after being confined for two months in hospital, when I came out I really did see my life from a different perspective. Of course, I was still doing things wrong in life — for starters, spending too much on unnecessary clothing. But what I realized, to my surprise, was that I actually had a life. This, I hadn't even contemplated before, but the reality was that I did have opportunities. I did have a future, even though for twenty years I had done very little. My future for the first time appeared bright, and this gave me the biggest anxiety attack I've had yet.

The thought of getting on with my life was all a bit too much for me, and I became fearful that I would fail eventually. Fear of failing meant that I didn't even try certain things.

It was then that I decided to look for work again. I had not done that for many years. I went on a few interviews and was overlooked. Then, I decided to work on my CV, which I have done, and I am still currently applying for work while writing this book.

This was one step in the right direction, but my struggles with anxiety did not stop there. Every morning, when I woke up, I felt anxious and fearful. This was my first feeling before the day had even begun. I questioned what I was going to do with the day, and that made me anxious. It only subsided during the afternoon, and then it would lay off until the evening, when it would eventually come back again.

I found that I'd be more anxious if I had missed breakfast in the morning. So, I try to make breakfast every day and change things around to make it interesting, as it helps start the day off on the right foot. Like exercise, breakfast activates the brain again and brings those happy feelings back. Providing your brain with food helps you process your thoughts and then realize what you are going to do with your day. The best thing I've found to quell my anxiety is to find things to do.

For many days, I remember myself being inactive and despondent. I would lie in bed without getting dressed, as I was too afraid to leave the bedroom, and would loiter around the house with no purpose, which would only increase my levels of anxiety. Sometimes I had no local supplies and nothing to fuel any energy that I needed. Moping around the home had become a soft comfort for me when I was too frightened to leave because of agoraphobia.

I would dwell on things that now seem so unnecessary. I would stay cooped up and hardly talk to anyone. This was sometimes a daily or weekly basis; I would have no one to talk to. This has such a damaging effect on your mental health. Social interaction is important, and when you are not interacting with anyone, it means that you are self-sabotaging, focusing only on yourself and your problems every day. The repetitiveness of this brings you into a state of depression quicker than if you were in regular contact with people.

Talking about other things apart from your problems in life also helps. It's surprising how much fear can build up once you are left to your own devices. That's why it's so important to make an effort to go out or have that conversation at home. Interacting with as many people as you can helps alleviate fear and de-stresses you in the long term. Making the point to be sociable can change your day tremendously from having an anxious day full of fear to a more meaningful, pleasant day.

Being physically able to go out by getting a bus pass or driving can make all the difference. It just means you are ready when the opportunity knocks. You can get out, and you do not have to go to the same place all the time. You can do something different with your life if you are just a little bit more adventurous.

Opening up your senses to adventure is one way of meeting your dreams. It stops you from stagnating and allows you to live beyond your fears. Change the driving force in your life; the one that tells you that you have to do the same things all the time, even if the effects are not productive. It seems like you remain with a staple of bad choices that take you no further than the front door.

When you have anxiety, you have to make a

conscious effort to be happy at all costs. Anything that brings joy and laughter into your life should be encouraged.

Then there are your achievements in life. No one gets to any stage in life without achieving anything. There is always something that they have achieved whether this was top-notch grades at A levels, or GCSEs, or a degree. It could be a short course that you attended or a longer course, either way it matters. Completing it is still an achievement that you should be proud of.

Friendship is also a great achievement. You should be grateful for your network of friends, no matter how small it is right now. Even if you only have one friend, be thankful. Be grateful for your family members as well, especially when they are alive. Now I know that sounds strange to say, but too often we can take family members for granted, and it's only when they move away or are physically not here anymore that we take the time to appreciate them.

Gratitude said in prayer is something that reminds us that there have been better days, and we can get back to them, and even create better days still, in the future. You just have to wish for better things in your life. Remember to be grateful for what you have already — be grateful for having a front door to come home to, your own house, or a space that is yours, whether you own it or rent it. Be grateful that you still have a brain, one that is still functional and reminds you to do what is necessary.

CHAPTER 7 — MAKING GOOD

All our dreams can come true, if we have the courage to pursue them.

– Walt Disney

There are so many little things to be grateful for — like the fact that you are breathing right now, whether it is shallow breath or a deep breath — you are alive and are conscious of the fact. Be thankful that you have some money in the bank and although it may not be a lot, it's still better than nothing at all. Be thankful that you have those occasional lie-ins to rejuvenate yourself. Be grateful that you can cook a healthy meal to sustain your body. Be grateful that you can go out and exercise whenever you need to; you can even wake up and decide to go for a run that day. Be thankful that you can head over to your nearest gym, or go swimming for that matter.

The freedom that you have is immense! It is only fear — again — that stops you from entertaining any one of these things. The fear of breaking a routine is harmful to you, because staying inside, lying in bed for too long, and worrying about unnecessary things, does you no good. Gratitude brings the joy factor back into your life. Listing all the things that you are grateful for will help you when you are having your bad days, and when you're feeling of fear overwhelms you, you can send it to the cooler. That's right — send it straight to the cooler with all of its associated symptoms.

Fear is only here to strip joy of its tasks — joy is something that you should carry around with you at all times. As mentioned, I struggle with anxiety from the time I wake up in the morning, until the early evening.

There seems to be a regular worry that I have, and every day that I am worried about something, the intensity of it gets bigger as the worry increases — this is how I function. Whether it subsides a little or not, each day starts with the same amount of worry and concern. It fogs my brain, and repeats itself as angst and a burning sensation in my heart, accompanied by sweats and more brain fog. Shivers and numbness follow, and by then it is hard to function like a normal human.

> *Develop a habit called courage to get rid of fear*
> *— Tony Robbins*

When these insurmountable feelings occur, the first thing to do is to break the cycle, perhaps with a hot drink, like a cup of tea or coffee. Somehow, the drinking motion breaks the numbness. Then, if you can get something to eat, it is even better. I find porridge is an easy thing to make and eat. It gives immediate nutrition and helps you feel better instantly.

There are a variety of things that you can do to break the habits that cause anxiety. Anything that takes you outside of yourself for a few minutes will definitely help you. The thing about anxiety is that it's a 'thinking state'. The way we think about things, the way our mind processes everyday life, is what causes us to experience anxiety. So, refrain from negative thoughts daily — getting outside of negative thoughts, and a negative spiral of thinking, is super important. Although, changing negative thoughts to positive ones is easier said than done, which is why pessimistic thinking becomes a habit. As a result, it's important to make a note of our daily habits and rituals.

Suppose you start the day like I often do, with negative thoughts — saying things like, I am not worthy of such a thing, or I do not deserve this or that in my life. The funny thing is that if you had a friend that spoke to you this way, you would get rid of that friend or do away with such a person for good. Yet you do this to yourself continuously! You are — at times — the creator of your own unhappiness. So, what you need to do is to imagine life without these daily, toxic interruptions. You have to teach yourself not to accept them anymore, even when a little doubt creeps in that can lead you into a downward spiral of negative feelings, as this can soon grow and get out of control, and it's hard to know where to go when this happens to you.

Self-doubt is like a leech; it is the worst thing for your self-confidence. If we disbelieve in ourselves, it's going to be very difficult to convince people to believe in us and our ability. It drains us of all of our self-confidence and affects the way we interact with each other. But as mentioned before, there are negative spiralling habits that you have to kick out at the same time. These are the habits that keep us subdued. It is here where we lose all hope for the future. It promotes the uneasiness in our stomachs, prevents us from finding our true self, can lead us to severe depression and, if untreated, can immobilize us.

You should consider taking vitamin supplements to help give your body a boost and improve your brain function. Having regular meals will also help — this is all basic advice, but it is essential to your wellbeing.

Coping with anxiety every day is very difficult, and the

amount of people suffering from anxiety is growing daily. Maybe it is because we are more aware of what it is now. Every day I hear of another coping technique, and I note it down, much of which has already been covered in this book. Some swear by yoga as a way to shift anxiety. Others go running, as that also helps soothe the mind and body. Some base their lives on eating well and following healthy regimes by using fruit and vegetables to make smoothies that help boost the immune system. A healthy and balanced diet helps fight against tiredness and lethargy, and is another viable coping mechanism.

Whatever your exercise routine is, it seems if you have one, it can alter your mental health. As long as you have a regime, it will make you feel better. Some people prefer running on an open road. This can take you out of yourself for a while. It's scenic, and you can do it on your own. Raising your stamina increases your heart rate, and the blood flow to your head. It's a great way of starting your day, relieving your stress straight away.

It's also always good to have stable and consistent sleeping habits. At the moment, my sleeping habits are not very good. I tend to take my phone to my bed at night and have difficulty going to sleep, so waking up can be a struggle at times. But a better habit is to go to bed by ten and wake up around six. This is a good eight-hour sleep.

What I tend to do is try to wind down early, setting off to my bedroom at around eight, which is too early for sleep but not too early to prepare your body for sleep. I try to get even more hours of sleep under my belt, but it does not work out most nights as it feels that I have not completely rested. I am therefore exhausted in the mornings and do not have time to go for a run, which would help my mood.

Poor sleeping patterns are not good for your mental health, and they can result in more anxiety throughout the day. So, as it's imperative to have good sleep hygiene, try to remember all the things you should do before bed. Make sure that the temperature is right for you, make sure the curtains in your bedroom block out the light, and that you are not watching too much television before going to bed, nor staying on your phone, and lastly, that you are not having caffeine-rich drinks before bed.

Having a shower or bath before you go to bed helps to de-stress and loosen the muscles that might have been tense all day, and this is a much better alternative to coffee of tea.

Having erratic sleeping patterns can cause anxiety to creep back into your life as sleep deprivation is one of its key triggers. So, It's important to calm down just before you go to bed. Doing things like meditation and yoga before bed has been proven to reduce anxiety levels and promote a better rest all around. Going to bed too early, when you are not tired enough, can also produce poor sleep, but something soothing — like reading a book before bedtime — can help the onset of sleep, and a better one at that.

The aim is to try and get eight hours of sleep, and getting at least six hours of solid sleep is desirable. The more uninterrupted sleep you get at night, the more rested and fresher you will be during the daytime.

When you are tired in the daytime, it means you are not acting on optimum potential or drive. You do things half-heartedly and without much energy or concentration. That is why it is important to be fresh and energized during the day. In order to reap the opportunities of the day, you cannot be tired from the night before. Therefore, it's important to undergo a regular nighttime routine, because good sleep hygiene results in good mental health.

Self-awareness is also quite important. Once you can attribute tiredness to lack of sleep, you can do some of the things that I've mentioned earlier to promote a good night's sleep. Of course, tiredness can come about because of overworking and poor diet. If you are firing on all cylinders every day without any rest incorporated in your day, you will either collapse or burnout. You are also far more likely to get a cold and become ill — everything in moderation is necessary.

You still need to work, but if you limit your working hours to 30 hours a week, it's a good start. Equally, if you are not working and you have a period where you find it a struggle to get up in the morning, prepare your breakfast and main meals. But even if you are not working, you need to get yourself into a routine, and I believe a six-hour day gives you the opportunity to do something constructive in the week. And be sure to organize your time effectively. Take an art class or do something voluntary if you have time, but just do *something*. Otherwise, you can get to the stage where you are tired most of the time with no ambitions, no nutrients, and no prospects. If this is the case, then you need to make a change because this is the kind of lifestyle that attracts fear, and if you do things to attract fear, you are shutting out the other good things that would bring a better change, like an opportunity at love, abundance, hope, joy, and clarity.

CHAPTER 8 — FOLLOWING ON

If we did all the things we are capable of, we would literally astound ourselves.

– Thomas Edison

A support system is essential for recovery. Early intervention from professionals and all care givers will most likely achieve a speedier recovery. There is much ignorance around mental health, and this lack of understanding has helped the stigma of mental health to continue, and has stopped people from seeking treatment. Things are thankfully changing with education, work and personal stories, like that of the Duke and Duchess of Cambridge, and Prince Harry and Meghan. We need to address the problems of young people to help them cope with their feelings now, rather than later.

If you are continuously attracting fear, you will find yourself weary and demotivated, and without a desire to do anything, be anywhere, or see anyone. This method of attracting more and more fear into your life is toxic, making us establish fear as our deafault setting. This vibration is not healthy, and it can only hinder you.

Changing your vibrational energy is what you need to do next. Invite all that is in the positive flow, all that is good, all that is loving and nurturing, all that is compassionate, all that is wholesome, and try introducing all these things into your life by shutting the door on fear permanently. This is something that you need to practice daily. Try making good vibrations every time something comes into your energy path that isn't wholesome. Flag it up as an intruder in your life and banish it for good. Do not just accept it, and do not convince yourself that you need it in any way or form.

This is an addictive behavioural pattern, and the addiction is to pain and misery. It does not matter that you have been here before with this experience, but it has to be said that you no longer want this intrusion in your life. So, we have to stamp it out firmly and forever. Why would you accept pain and misery in your life as a way of living? You should not accept it by choice but you are doing so by constantly feeding the fear in your life. This enters you into a dialogue with misery and unhappiness.

When you enter into this dialogue, it is one-sided, and the onslaught is terrible   attacking you from left and right, so that you do not know which way to turn and you have fear infiltrating from all angles. It's like a meteor attack on your whole being. But rather than accepting it as a defeat, you have to do something about it. Letting fear into your life is only a negative spiral that keeps twisting and mutating. It undermines your confidence and brings on anxiety and depression.

It pays to have healthy conversations stating that you are not anxious, you are not depressed, and you are not fearful — that's the key. By replacing these words every day, you will become a whole new person once again. So, when you say you feel fear all over your body, you resume to learn to change the dialogue — I feel joy all over my body, I feel abundance, I feel clarity, I feel at ease.

Every day that you have a negative thought — such as, I'm not worthy, I am sad, or I do not deserve to live — replace it with positive thoughts — I am everything that I need to be, I am all I need to be at the moment, all I need is here, I am courageous, I am a trailblazer, I am capable of doing much more than I realize, I am steadfast, I am enough, I am more than I ever was, I am grateful, I am loved, I am a soldier and I'll keep fighting, I am resilient, I can cope with adversaries, I can be better than I am now — any of these thoughts help.

With the right training, you can overcome the impossible. You can look fear in the eyes and say — you are not part of me, you have no control over my life, you will not outline how I live in the future, you will not dictate my needs anymore, you are but a passing emotion, you have no place in my life.

I have replaced all of my negative emotions with positive emotions, and this has come in handy in terms of acknowledging how far I have come. And I have come a long way. I have uprooted myself from the quagmire and taken myself out of situations where I would be stagnant. I have taken the challenge to learn more about my emotions and understand how to combat the negative feelings head-on. They are only here temporarily, and I now know how to disperse them, how to stop them from taking so much of my time.

When I'm feeling low, I now know not to indulge in feelings of despair and despondency, I now know that it's better to let the feeling ride and think of it as a temporary phase. And it will not last very long, especially if I hold my ground. I have taken the challenge to combat these negative feelings head-on by sorting them into groups as they often follow certain categories.

The first set of negative thoughts goes like this — I am not worth it, I do not have anything to bring to the table, I do not have any skills, I am a loser with no prospects, I am useless, I am unlovable.

How does one feel worthy enough in one's self to get rid of these feelings or implications that you are not enough? The best way to do this is by remembering that these are just blanket statements that do not make any sense. You choose to believe the lie when you are having an off day, or you are feeling less confident, which is not helpful.

We believe all sorts of things when we are hard on ourselves. Sometimes, we are our own worst enemy. The negative self-talk is something that takes practise to disregard, and if you are used to having it all the time, it's time to put an end to it. You would never put up with this type of talk from a friend or someone close. A friend knows when you are feeling down or having a bad day, and they are there to build you up and make you feel better about things. A friend listens constructively and would not entertain the onslaught of negative vibes that you have given yourself every day. It's not a balanced view of yourself.

When you get into states of depression and anxiety, a friend or family member is what you need at times to bring you out of it. But the key is to learn how not to get into it in the first place. And if you do find yourself in it, the best way to counter it is to be kind to yourself. Carry out some appropriate self-talk that helps you with your thought process.

Let's face it — you really had no one at your back. You are unlikely to want to hear negative streams coming from within you or anywhere else. These negative emotions wash over you like waves, and you have drowned in them. They are everywhere, all-consuming, and you are just trying to breathe and keep your head above water.

The whole purpose of these thoughts is self-destruction. They leave you feeling diseased and off kilter — you end up wanting and clinging to these emotions more because deep down, you think the alternative will be more painful, and this is a pain you are used to. This pain is familiar, and almost comforting.

You forget the fact that these emotions cause real pain, and that without these emotions, there is no pain. But the addictive nature of this pulls us deeper and deeper into its claws, and sooner or later you are experiencing negative emotions, when you should be spending your time experiencing positive emotions and getting rid of any conflict that you might be experiencing.

The hardest thing to do is to leave the old life behind. It comes as part of a realization that it is important to find an authentic and ultimate purpose in your life. It's something that has to be sought-after at every waking opportunity. Living a more purposeful life and having one that has healthy boundaries is the key. It is one where you are your best friend in every area of life. Nurture that inner best friend and give them the tools necessary to help you in your recovery. Let it be a pep talk that you regularly need! What would you say to yourself if you are going through a patch of demotivation and despondency, for example? Would you not advise yourself to take things one step at a time? Manage them into sizeable chunks? Well, you can do it. It just takes a little time and effort.

What if you are not feeling confident? The only way out is to practice, practice, and practice again — until you are confident. Every journey starts with the first step. And you must muster the courage to take that first step. Change is bound to happen, but you have to want it badly enough to get anywhere in life. Anything is better than living the life you are currently living, and you have to believe that — this is the first step on the road to recovery.

The next step is to have healthy habits. This involves getting rid of everything that is not good for you anymore and replacing them with healthy habits. For example, if you are used to skipping breakfast in the morning, make it your task is to have breakfast every morning, and also to make the eating process enjoyable by introducing new foods to your diet.

Healthy habits cover a range of things, like getting up in the morning at a reasonable time, making time to exercise, and clearing your space and mind of unnecessary clutter. Free your mind up for new possibilities by getting rid of everything unnecessary in your life.

There are activities like Feng Shui that can help you de-clutter. The best thing to do is to start in a corner and keep at it until you have got rid of everything you do not need in that corner, and afterwards go around the room tackling each corner. Then, hit the big space and gradually get rid of everything that you do not need, or anything that doesn't bring you joy.

It can take time, but one idea a friend gave me was that reducing paperwork also works sometimes. Reduce your paperwork so that only 10% of it is left. This seems achievable now that we live in such a technological world, as we do not have to get rid of everything we need, but we can still reduce this physical paper clutter.

Then, there was another example of getting rid of 29 items a day for nine days. They could be cracked old mugs or clothing items which you never wear. Anything that you have not used, especially in the last ten years. Just get rid of it or give it to a charity shop. It will be so worth it when you realise you have more space for other things. This is unimaginably freeing and creates a scope for further creative ideas.

You will have more time to spend on the things that you love doing by being quicker and more efficient when it comes to choosing your items of clothing. It will be easier to clean the house or apartment once all the clutter has gone. If you are disciplined with it, it should not take a lot of time. And in no time at all, your head clutter will also dissipate.

It's so important to have less clutter in your life; it helps your brain focus on what is crucial, which then helps with what you actually want to do. A cleaner environment helps the brain think more clearly. It also helps with sleep problems, as it is easier to sleep when your surroundings are in order — otherwise, you may be constantly triggering your anxiety.

Now that you are happy with your newly decluttered space, remember to save your money and reduce wasteful expenses. If you purchase new clothes, but keep the old and unused ones in the wardrobe, you are not moving forward, you are creating more of a problem. So, contruct a system that works for you.

There is nothing worse than spending time buying more stuff without accounting for what you already have. And when you buy new things, they have to go with what you already have, or you are wasting precious money again. This is money that could go towards a holiday or some other recreational activity during times of stress — it's nice to remember that you have some savings for a rainy day.

By only buying things that you really need, you learn self-control in many areas of your life. It's a good path to follow and you will live on a far better footing than before.

Once you have mastered this habit, you need to follow it religiously — know your limitations, set boundaries for living, have a healthy attitude towards money, learn how to spend appropriately, learn how to offer solutions to money problems, and learn to prioritize. It is always good to be conscious of how much money you have and what you are spending that money on, especially when you know that it would be better to spend it on nutritional food than on endless outfits you may wear once in your life.

Be sure to fuel your body first before you attempt anything else in life. You should also always have nutritional meals as they will elate your mood, and you will feel better after it.

The habit of buying fresh fruit and vegetables is one that needs to be practised a lot. There are lots of supermarkets selling fresh fruit and vegetables. So, there is no excuse to not organize a trip once a week. It is definitely a healthy habit worth keeping up. You are less likely to be run down or unwell, and you will also sleep better with the right nutrition, when you make a routine out of it. It guarantees that whatever food you are having, you are moving forwards not backwards.

Another great habit is to prepare meals in advance. Make larger portions and split them down into smaller portions, so that you can eat them in rotation. It's another way to save money as it also ensures that you are eating adequately. This fuels your body and makes you function better as a human being. Maintaining a routine like this is extremely desirable. It helps ward off ailments and keeps the body functioning normally. The levels of fruit and vegetables in your diet should be high, as they make you feel healthier and better — and if you feel physically better, your outlook will be better, leaving you with less time to be anxious or depressed. A balanced diet is a win-win situation; it's healthy for your body and it's healthy for your mind.

So, the idea is to keep practicing healthy habits. You will immediately see that a healthy diet has a direct effect on the body and hence how you feel — better health results in a better you!

We spoke about good sleep, good hygiene, and making sure that you are ready to go to bed. Try to exercise or take a bath before you go to bed, as these are healthy habits that help you to relax and cleanse your mind. Another habit is to be mindful of what you are thinking — especially paying attention to the negative thought patterns that come up daily in the morning, and then again late in the evening. Replacing these thoughts with positive affirmations is a great habit to have.

So, de-cluttering, good nutrition and a sleeping routine, are just three healthy habits that can take you on the road to recovery.

Nutrition is incredibly important, and it is imperative to have three meals a day, every day; it's a good way of reducing weight, and it provides the body with necessary nutrients.

Try looking into sleep hygiene to make sure that your body gets the requirement of rest it needs to store all the nutrients in the body, and to be able to continue functioning optimally.

The more you venture outside your four walls the more you mood will be lifted. Moreover, you can take inspiration from your new surroundings.

And to reiterate, toxic self talk is no use to anyone. List all the qualities that make you unique and loveable and challenge negative thoughts by doing something new. Most of all, try to have fun.

Positive self-talk, along with the following, will make you feel better:-

Listen to cheerful music
Make morning schedules
Exercise in the open air
Live one day at a time
Do something that brings you joy
Go swimming
Embrace positive thoughts
Acknowledge your accomplishments
Have a good laugh
Go for a walk
De-clutter

The term psychological myopia refers to repetitive, negative thoughts based around core beliefs, like 'nothing ever works out for me'. This makes you stuck seeing things one way, when there is a plethora of perspectives.

Visualising happy memories instead of replaying painful memories is another way forward. Learn to stop telling yourself nothing good will ever happen.

It is all about providing alternatives for yourself, and getting used to self-affirming thoughts that remove the continuous negative self-talk that brings us into a spiral of despair and anxiety.

So, to take that leap of faith to maintain a positive attitude and keep this mental habit going despite whatever is happening around you. For it is the positive thinking that can now keep you constantly moving forward, rather than being stuck in a negative mental state.

It may, of course, be discomforting at first, but it takes perseverance — complete perseverance. It will seem easier to stick with depression and despondency and all the negative thoughts that come with it, which put you down every day.

It's easier to be in this state as it is familiar — you are used to the onslaught from the enemy within yourself — with your thoughts and expectations that torment you. That's why if you can switch it around to positive thinking, it gets better overall. Having suffered anxiety, I know how hard it is to turn it around. Staying focused on the positives is outside of your comfort zone, and even though it's uncomfortable, it's what you know, and you can sit with this feeling.

But you need to know that it is okay to think that there is something better for you out there. Indeed, there *is* something better for you out there. Something that will make you feel more positive and, therefore, will allow for positive things to happen to you. This mindset is something that can impact every area of your life for the better — yet we have a fear of it. But you have to turn the corner with this, surprise yourself with new thinking that will take on all past thinking patterns, and challenge them so that they become positive in every way possible. It will happen especially when you are feeling low, unloved, and lonely. This is why it's good to have a mindset that changes this feeling.

Looking at the positives — in all situations — alleviates a lot of pain and heartache. We have got to be our own best friend. Instead of thinking 'what are the ways I did it wrong?', change it to 'what are the ways I did it right?'

You should not continue to feel bad about your situation and your life, believing that you will never get a partner, or that you will never find someone again. Because then, all the subsequent thoughts — that no one will ever want you again, that you are not worthy of being loved, that you are not interesting enough, that you do not look great compared to others — will affect your self-esteem, and again this is your internal voice saying it. It's no one else's internal dialogue that is constantly lowering *your* self-worth.

These thoughts are damaging because they do not beat you down once, they do it continuously. So, even when you have a little bit of self-esteem, it is yourself that is your enemy again. When you are finding it hard to remain positive, you change the dialogue because it is a learned behaviour. Behaviour that is so natural to you that it forms part of your daily pattern; it becomes second nature. But it is so wrong and harmful for your psyche and your wellbeing. And the destructive effect that it has on your daily interactions is obvious, meaning that you have fewer than normal. And the ones you do have lack meaning or purpose because they are drowned out by this negative cycle that you are finding difficult to break.

But I implore you to persevere, and if you are struggling with anxiety, I hope some of the techniques mentioned here do help you.

When you are feeling anxious, it's great to be able to distract yourself with something else. Something that can really grasp your attention in ways that your anxiety cannot — that queasy feeling in your stomach or that shortness of breath *can* be eradicated. It is important to relax, even to meditate, to take your thoughts away from yourself and stop worrying about things that might not even happen. Choose instead to plan an active, fulfilled life where you can make time for fun activities regularly.

This will stop you from feeling needlessly uptight and reduce stress levels substantially. The key is always to reduce the stress that makes you feel uncomfortable. Sometimes doing less can help with stress levels.

So, think of alternative ways of relaxing when you start to feel stressed out —imagine yourself sitting on a beach, walking in the woods, relaxing in a swimming pool, or anything that takes you to a happy place. And if you find it difficult to relax straight away, take a deep breath, and practise your breathing — breathe in for four counts, then out on for four counts. Deep breaths fill the body up with oxygen and the more oxygen the brain gets, the better. I know it's a struggle sometimes, but there are definite habit-breaking techniques that we can learn and instil within our daily routines.

Hiding, hesitating, and being hypercritical are some of the ways we react to situations when influenced by self-doubt. When self-doubt comes into play, sometimes you hesitate, which inevitably stops you from doing something you want to do. Hesitation leaves you numb and in a somewhat paralysing state. It is torture through self-doubt, which is why you have to learn to not hesitate.

Hiding is another problem to be avoided. You may hide behind the thoughts or actions that you feel you have to take, or simply avoid doing what is necessary. This does not help anything and also leads to procrastination, which feeds your self-doubt.

Being hypercritical of your plans means that you are always talking yourself out of doing things by saying that you are not good enough and you might not be able to cope. You may have pessimistic thoughts that you are doing things wrong, you are not getting the right results, or you cannot possibly achieve anything. (Source unknown internet)

These self-limiting beliefs are not only frustrating, but they are also the fire that burns behind self-doubt. The relentless negative talk — which convinces you that you are not capable, you will never be successful, you will never achieve anything, among others — is so debilitating. These thoughts are the ones that need to be eradicated. All self-doubt does is propagate fear and anxiety, or worse, it takes you to the point of no return. Trying to overcome this feeling is never easy, but it is necessary. Learn to put a safety plan in place — I will learn to calm myself, I will call…, I will go to…— otherwise, you retain the glum outlook on life and have no hope for the future. You are continuously battling woe, which is a tremendous uphill struggle, but you can opt out of it. Because of it, you are unable to think beyond the negative options. Yet, there are so many possibilities once you have retrained your thinking, you only need to trust your new mindset rather than procrastinating in fear. You could be planning your authentic life; a life that holds possibilities, a life that values your contributions and efforts, a life where you do not have to question whether you are doing the right thing. Ultimately, you are always doing the right thing, and you should be aiming for results now.

But nothing is going to change unless you review your circumstances, take ownership of your actions and behaviours, and ask yourself where you are going and what you are doing. Your life is no one's responsibility but yours.

Remember your responsibility to make reasonable efforts towards feeling better. You must be able to look at your past with a sense of contentment and look forward to a fulfilled future.

As of now, you are learning to make your life worthwhile, filling it up with things, rather than leaving things to fester and getting nothing done.

Waiting till you feel like it is never going to change you, you have to go for what you deserve in your life or what you truly desire. Keep the momentum, don't go by how you feel, commit to do it anyway.

— *Tony Robbins*

If you can:-
Turn pain into power
Turn fear into courage
Turn difficulties into determination

If you do these things, you will find that you have achieved more than most, and you will be on your way to having a fulfilled and happy life.

The only thing you have in life is will. Our habits control our lives. Stretch your life, name your standards, and change your life. Remember healthy habits and rituals make it real.
— *Tony Robbins*

There is a far greater life somewhere, so be ready to have access to it. And remember, nothing succeeds like a positive mind-set!

USEFUL ORGANISATIONS
AND MOTIVATORS

HAY HOUSE
SAMARITANS
PREMIER LIFELINE
SONIA CHOQUETTE
MUCHELLEB
FREDERIC BROS
AUDREY COYNE
KELLY STAMPS
BI-POLAR UK
TONY ROBBINS
GRANT CARDONE

VIKTOR FRANKL INSTITUTE
THE CHARTERHOUSE CLINIC
THE MINDED INSTITUTE
EXTRA RESOURCES

getselfhelp.co.uk
thedecider.org.uk

Near Restful Waters-
Reflections on Psalm 23
Sr. Josephine Walsh, D.H.S

ABOUT THE AUTHOR

Nicola Espeut lives in North London. She has completed voluntary work that has taken her to Namibia, Nepal, and Cotopaxi, and she still volunteers in the UK.

She is an avid singer-songwriter and poet, too.

Contact her at nespeut@hotmail.com

All I Need Is here is an inspirational book that takes you on a journey out of the darkness and into the light. It encourages you to believe that all the answers to your troubles are within you. It is about one woman's coping strategies to meet the excruciating demands of anxiety and depression. It gives insight into the inner demons and inner critique, and the techniques you can use to stop yourself falling into the quagmire of despair. It is a fast-paced, interactive book that gives hope for a debilitating condition.

Lightning Source UK Ltd.
Milton Keynes UK
UKHW041100110722
405686UK00001B/50